# HEALTH CARE COST,

# QUALITY, AND OUTCOMES

## ISPOR BOOK OF TERMS

Editors

MARC L. BERGER, MD

KERSTIN BINGEFORS, PhD

EDWIN C. HEDBLOM, PharmD

CHRIS L. PASHOS, PhD

GEORGE W. TORRANCE, PhD

Managing Editor

MARILYN DIX SMITH, RPh, PhD

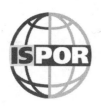

INTERNATIONAL SOCIETY FOR PHARMACOECONOMICS
AND OUTCOMES RESEARCH

Ordering information is available by calling ISPOR at 609-219-0773, or visit the ISPOR Web site at www.ispor.org.

Library of Congress Control Number: 2003113121
ISBN: 0-9743289-0-1

# Contents

# Contributors

ABBOTT, THOMAS, PhD, *Merck & Co*, West Point, PA, USA
ALEMAO, EVO, MS, *Merck & Co*, Whitehouse Station, NJ, USA
ALTHIN, RIKARD, PhD, *Pharmacia Ltd*, Yorkshire, United Kingdom
BELL, HANAN, PhD, Seattle, WA, USA
BERGER, WOLFGANG, PhD, *Merck KGaA*, Darmstadt, Germany
BERZON, RICK, DrPH, *Boehringer Ingelheim Pharmaceuticals*, Ridgefield, CT, USA
BOBULA, JOEL, MA, *Wyeth*, Ayerest Research, Philadelphia, PA, USA
BOLINDER, BJORN, BA, *Aventis Pharmaceuticals*, Bridgewater, NJ, USA
BOSE, UDAY KUMAR, MSc, BSc, *Aventis Pharma Ltd*, Kent, United Kingdom
BOULANGER, LUKE, MA, *Boston Health Economics*, Waltham, MA, USA
BUDHIARSO, ISMAIL, MA, *Health Research Associates*, Seattle, WA, USA
BUSHNELL, DON, MA, *Health Research Associates*, Seattle, WA, USA
CAPPELLERI, JOSEPH, PhD, MPH, MS, *Pfizer Inc*, Groton, CT, USA
CARO, JAIME, MD, *Caro Research Institute*, Concord, MA, USA
CARTER, JEAN, PhD, PharmD, *University of Montana*, Missoula, MT, USA
CHIOU, CHIUN-FANG, PhD, *Zynx Health Inc*, Beverly Hills, CA, USA
CLARK, MARY ANN, MHA, *Boston Scientific*, Natick, MA, USA
CRAMER, JOYCE, *Yale University School of Medicine*, New Haven, CT, USA
CROWN, WILLIAM, PhD, MA, *The MEDSTAT Group*, Cambridge, MA, USA
DUBOIS, DOMINIQUE, MD, *Johnson & Johnson Pharmaceutical Services*, Beerse, Belgium
DUH, MEI-SHENG, MPH, ScD, *Analysis Group*, Boston, MA, USA
EDELMAN LEWIS, BARBARA, PhD, MHA, *AstraZeneca*, Wilmington, DE, USA
EINARSON, THOMAS, PhD, *University of Toronto*, Toronto, Canada
ERICKSON, PENNIFER, PhD, *O.L.G.A.*, State College, PA, USA
FARQUHAR, IRENE, PhD, *Health Services Solutions*, Columbia, MD, USA
FENWICK, ELISABETH, PhD, *University of York*, York, United Kingdom
FLANDERS, SCOTT, PhD, *TAP Pharmaceuticals*, Lake Forest, IL, USA
FRICKE, FRANK-ULRICH, PhD, *Fricke & Pirk Gmb*, Nuremberg, Germany
GARRISON, LOU, PhD, *Roche Pharmaceuticals*, Basel, Switzerland
GIRTS, TAMMY, PharmD, MS, *Boehringer Ingelheim Pharmaceuticals*, Ridgefield, CT, USA
GRAUER, DENNIS, PhD, RPh, MS, *University of Kansas*, Kansas City, KS, USA
HALPERN, MICHAEL, MD, PhD, *Exponent*, Alexandria, VA, USA
HARRIS, CRYSTAL, RPh, PharmD, *VA Cooperative Studies*, Albuquerque, NM, USA
HEISSEL, ARNE, PhD, *Ethicon Endo-Surgery*, Norderstedt, Germany
HESS, GREGORY, MD, MBA, *Drexel University*, Wayne, PA, USA
HOBBS, CONNIE, *RTI Health Solutions*, Research Triangle Park, NC, USA
HUTTON, JOHN, BPhil, BSc, *MEDTAP International*, London, United Kingdom
ISACSON, DAG, PhD, *Uppsala University*, Uppsala, Sweden
IRISH, WILLIAM, PhD, MSc, *RTI Health Solutions*, Research Triangle Park, NC, USA
JIMENEZ, JAVIER, MD, MPH, *AstraZeneca Farmaceutica*, Madrid, Spain
JOHANNES, ERNST, MD, *NV Organon*, Oss City, The Netherlands

JOHNSON, IAN, BSc, *Thomson Interphase*, Macclesfield, United Kingdom

JOISH, VIJAY, MS, *Pharmacotherapy Outcomes Research Center*,
   Salt Lake City, UT, USA

KEININGER, DOROTHY, MS, *MAPI Values*, Boston, MA, USA

KLEIN, ERIC, PharmD, *Eli Lilly and Co*, Indianapolis, IN, USA

KLING, CARSTEN, MBA, *Mediconomics GmbH*, Hannover, Germany

KONG, SHELDON, PhD, *Merck & Co*, Whitehouse Station, NJ, USA

KORELITZ, JAMES, PhD, *Westat*, Rockville, MD, USA

KOZMA, CHRIS, PhD, West Columbia, SC, USA

LEE, JEFF, PharmD, *Allergan*, Irvine, CA, USA

LIERMAN, WALTER, PhD, *HWS, Inc*, USA

LILJAS, BENGT, PhD, *AstraZeneca*, Lund, Sweden

LUCE, BRYAN, PhD, *MEDTAP International*, Bethesda, MD, USA

LYDICK, EVA, PhD, *LoveLace Clinic Foundation*, Albuquerque, NM, USA

LYU, RAMON, MS, *Merck & Co*, Whitehouse Station, NJ, USA

MANIADAKIS, NIKOLAOS, MSc, PhD, *Eli Lilly and Co*, Windlesham Surrey, United Kingdom

MANJUNATH, RANJANI, MSPH, *RTI Health Solutions*, Research Triangle Park, NC, USA

MARKSON, LEONA, ScD, *Merck & Co*, West Point, PA, USA

MARSH, WALLACE, PhD, MBA, *Nova Southeastern University*, Ft. Lauderdale, FL, USA

MARTIN, MONA, RN, MPA, *Health Research Associates*, Seattle, WA, USA

MARX, STEVEN, PharmD, PhD, MS, *Abbott Laboratories*, Abbott Park, IL, USA

McGHAN, WILLIAM, PharmD, PhD, *University of the Sciences in Philadelphia*, Philadelphia, PA, USA

MENZIN, JOSEPH, PhD, *Boston Health Economics*, Waltham, MA, USA

MERCHANT, SANJAY, MBA, PhD, *Bayer Pharmaceuticals Corporation*, West Haven, CT, USA

MEURER, STEVE, PhD, *St. Louis University*, St. Louis, MO, USA

MOTHERAL, BRENDA, RPh, MBA, PhD, *Express Scripts*, Maryland Heights, MO, USA

MYRIE, LESLIE, *RTI Health Solutions*, Research Triangle Park, NC, USA

NEIGHBORS, DEIRDRE, *RTI Health Solutions*, Research Triangle Park, NC, USA

O'HAGAN, ANTHONY, PhD, *University of Sheffield*, Sheffield, United Kingdom

PALTIEL, DAVID, PhD, *Yale School of Medicine*, New Haven, CT, USA

PAPATHEOFANIS, FRANK, MD, MPH, PhD, *UCSD*, San Diego, CA, USA

PICKARD, SIMON, PhD, *University of Illinois at Chicago*, Chicago, IL, USA

POSTMA, MAARTEN, PhD, *Groningen University Institute for Drug Exploration*, Groningen,
   The Netherlands

POULIOS, NICK, PhD, PhM, *Baxter Bioscience*, Westlake Village, CA, USA

PRIETO, LUIS, PhD, *Eli Lilly & Co*, Alcobendas (Madrid), Spain

RAISCH, DENNIS, RPh, PhD, *VA Cooperative Studies*, Albuquerque, NM, USA

REED, SHELBY, PhD, *United Kingdome Clinical Research Institute*, Durham, NC, USA

REED, PAMELA, DrPH, MPH, Allen, TX, USA

RICHTER, ANKE, PhD, *RTI Health Solutions*, Research Triangle Park, NC, USA

ROHRBACHER, RAINER, PhD, *HealthEcon Ltd*, Basel, Switzerland

ROTHMAN, MARGARET, PhD, *Johnson & Johnson Pharmaceutical Research*, Raritan, NJ, USA

RUBIO TERRES, CARLOS, MPEcon, *Aventis Pharma S.A.*, Madrid, Spain

RYCHLIK, REINHARD, MA, MD, PhD, *Institute of Empirical Health Economics*,
   Burscheid, Germany

SAMPSON, JEROME, MD, *Dept. of Veteran Affairs*, Alexandria, LA, USA
SCHUMOCK, GLEN, PHARMD, MBA, *University of Illinois at Chicago*, Chicago, IL, USA
SEAGRAVES, ARTHUR, RPH, *Merck & Co*, West Point, PA, USA
SEN, SHUVAYU, MS, *Merck & Co*, Whitehouse Station, NJ, USA
SENGUPTA, NISHAN, PHD, *Abbott Laboratories*, Abbott Park, IL, USA
SHELDON, ANDY, *TreeAge Software Inc.*, Williamstown, MA, USA
SHERRILL, BETH, *RTI International*, Research Triangle Park, NC, USA
SMITH, DAVID, PHD, *Kaiser Permanente Center for Health Research*, Portland, OR, USA
SONBO KRISTIANSEN, IVAR, MD, MPH, PHD, *University of Southern Denmark*,
    Odense, Denmark
SPRUILL, WILLIAM, PHARMD, *University of Georgia*, Athens, GA, USA
STANDAERT, BAUDOUIN, MD, *Amgen*, Brussels, Belgium
STEVENSON, JAMES, PHARMD, *University of Michigan Health Systems*, Ann Arbor, MI, USA
TEUTSCH, STEVEN, MD, MPH, *Merck & Co*, West Point, PA, USA
THOMAS, SIMU, PHD, *Novartis*, East Hanover, NJ, USA
THOMPSON, DAVID, PHD, *Innovus Research*, Medford, MA, USA
TORRANCE, GEORGE W., PHD, *McMaster University and Innovus Research*, Burlington,
    Ontario, Canada
TOUCHETTE, DANIEL, PHARMD, MA, *Oregon State University College of Pharmacy*,
    Portland, OR, USA
TRAN, HIEU, PHARMD, *Lake Erie College of Osteopathic Medicine*, Erie, PA, USA
TREGLIA, MICHAEL, PHD, *Pfizer Inc.*, Groton, CT, USA
TROTTER, JEFFREY, MM, *Ovation Research Group*, Highland Park, IL, USA
URQUHART, JOHN, MD, FRCP, *Maastricht University*, Maastricht, The Netherlands
VINKEN, ANGELA, MSC, *The Lewin Group*, Hoofddorp, The Netherlands
VOGENBERG, RANDY, RPH, PHD, *Aon Consulting*, Wellesley, MA, USA
WANG, JUNLING, MS, *University of Maryland*, Baltimore, MD, USA
WANG, YIZE RICHARD, MD, PHD, *AstraZeneca Pharmaceuticals*, Wilmington, DE, USA
WATSON, MARIA, PHD, *GlaxoSmithKline*, Research Triangle Park, NC, USA
WEIS, KATHLEEN, DRPH, PHD, MSN, ENP, *Pfizer*, New York, NY, USA
WILSON, MARCUS, PHARMD, *Health Core, Inc*, Newark, DE, USA
WILSON, LESLIE, PHD, MS, *University of California*, San Francisco, CA, USA
WITTRUP-JENSEN, KIM, BA, MSC, PHD, *Novo Nordisk A/S*, Bagsvaerd, Denmark
ZBROZEK, ARTHUR, MSC, MBA, *Wyeth Research*, Collegeville, PA, USA

# About ISPOR

THE INTERNATIONAL SOCIETY FOR PHARMACOECONOMICS AND OUT-COMES RESEARCH (ISPOR) is an international society organized to act as a scientific leader relevant to research in pharmacoeconomics, health outcomes assessment, and related issues of public policy. The Society represents health care researchers and practitioners including pharmacists, physicians, health economists, and other health care professionals involved in pharmacoeconomic analysis and health outcomes assessment.

The mission of ISPOR is to translate pharmacoeconomics and outcomes research into practice to ensure that society allocates scarce health care resources wisely, fairly, and efficiently.

The Society serves the public interest by the following means:
- Provides a global forum to facilitate the interchange of scientific knowledge in pharmacoeconomics and patient health outcomes;
- Facilitates and encourages communication among its members and with other research and educational groups, the communications media, and the general public by educating public and private agencies on the need for research in pharmacoeconomic and patient outcomes assessment;
- Acts as a global resource in forming public policy relevant to the pharmacoeconomics, health care outcomes assessment, and related issues of public concern;
- Promotes the science of pharmacoeconomics by assisting its members and providing such services as may be appropriate to conduct pharmacoeconomic and outcomes research, to support research applications in clinical practice, and to support scholarship and educational activities;
- Promotes cooperation and collaboration in pharmacoeconomics and outcomes assessment between all interested organizations, such as hospitals, managed care institutions, academia, health care providers, pharmaceutical companies, and government agencies;
- Represents the science of pharmacoeconomics and outcomes assessment before public and private bodies by identifying important issues concerning specific health care interventions, developing and publishing scientifically-based input for policy decisions, and making results of studies of pharmacoeconomics and health outcomes publicly available;
- Recognizes individual achievement in the field of pharmacoeconomics and outcomes research and;
- Fosters career growth and the development of its members for the betterment of the public health.

---

## INTERNATIONAL SOCIETY FOR PHARMACOECONOMICS AND OUTCOMES RESEARCH

3100 Princeton Pike   Building 3, Suite E   Lawrenceville, NJ 08648 USA

| PHONE | E-MAIL |
|---|---|
| 1-609-219-0773 | info@ispor.org |
| FAX | INTERNET |
| 1-609-219-0774 | www.ispor.org |

---

# Preface

THE INTERNATIONAL SOCIETY FOR PHARMACOECONOMICS AND OUTCOMES RESEARCH (ISPOR) is a nonprofit member-driven organization formed to promote the practice and science of pharmacoeconomics and health outcomes assessment. The mission of ISPOR is to promote research on the economic, clinical, and quality-of-life outcomes of health care interventions and to promote the translation of this research into information that health care decision-makers find useful.

THIS *HEALTH CARE COST, QUALITY, AND OUTCOMES: ISPOR BOOK OF TERMS* serves the mission of the Society. It includes over 100 entries covering more than 400 terms related to health care and the clinical, economic and patient-reported outcomes of that care as well as to the overall management and regulation of health care. Each entry focuses on a key term, briefly describes it, explains its use and value, describes issues related to it, and lists related terms and references.

*HEALTH CARE COST, QUALITY, AND OUTCOMES: ISPOR BOOK OF TERMS* builds on ISPOR's first publication, the *ISPOR LEXICON*™, to promote and facilitate greater understanding of health care outcomes research and its use in health care decisions. This book is targeted to health care professionals and decision-makers as well as to outcomes research practitioners and teachers. Accordingly, it serves multiple functions. It is a reference for the outcomes researcher, a user-friendly outcomes research lexicon and encyclopedia for the health care professional, and a comprehensive textbook for teachers of clinicians and student researchers.

*HEALTH CARE COST, QUALITY, AND OUTCOMES: ISPOR BOOK OF TERMS* would not have been possible without the numerous contributions by ISPOR members worldwide. Over 200 ISPOR members contributed to this book as authors or reviewers. Entries reflect perspectives of geographically diverse regions, including North America, Europe, Asia, Japan, and Australia, where knowledge of pharmacoeconomics and outcomes research is increasingly used in the health care decision-making process.

The editors gratefully acknowledge and thank ISPOR staff members Stephen L. Priori, Director of Publications, and Iman Nady, Coordinator of Publications, as well as Arne Heissel, PhD, 2001 ISPOR Fellow, for coordinating and facilitating the monograph solicitation and review process through final manuscript preparation.

We sincerely hope that *HEALTH CARE COST, QUALITY, AND OUTCOMES: ISPOR BOOK OF TERMS*, like the *ISPOR LEXICON*™, will help the practitioners of pharmacoeconomics and outcomes research and those who are users, consumers, or teachers of this research to improve communications, cooperation, and collaboration internationally in the comprehensive evaluation of health care outcomes.

Pharmacoeconomics and outcomes research will continue to evolve along with clinical practice and clinical research in general. We expect that future editions of *HEALTH CARE COST, QUALITY, AND OUTCOMES: ISPOR BOOK OF TERMS* will be needed to reflect the evolution of our field. In this regard, we welcome your feedback. Both general and specific comments as to how this book can be made more valuable are welcome.

*Editors*

MARC L. BERGER, MD
KERSTIN BINGEFORS, PhD
EDWIN C. HEDBLOM, PharmD
CHRIS L. PASHOS, PhD
GEORGE W. TORRANCE, PhD

*Managing Editor*

MARILYN DIX SMITH, RPh, PhD

# Bayesian Analysis

Frequentist Approach
Bayesian Analysis in Health
   Economics
Bayesian Approach

Posterior Interval
Posterior Distribution
Prior Distribution

## BRIEF DEFINITION

The Bayesian approach to statistics is fundamentally different from the approach that is traditionally taught to most students, which is now known as the **frequentist approach**. Statistical analysis conducted according to Bayesian principles would be called a **Bayesian analysis** (*see term*: Statistics in Pharmacoeconomics). Bayesian analysis involves the use of information that changes the likelihood or prior probability of an event to calculate a current risk that a person will experience that event. The Bayesian approach has been widely advocated for use in the solution of health economic problems, and there is a growing body of research using **Bayesian analysis in health economics**.

## EXPLANATION

The primary distinction between the Bayesian and frequentist approaches is that in the **Bayesian approach**, the unknown parameters in a statistical model are random variables. Accordingly, in a Bayesian analysis the parameters have probability distributions, whereas in frequentist analysis they are fixed but unknown quantities, and it is not permitted to make probability statements about them.

    This is puzzling to the layman, because a standard frequentist statement like a confidence interval certainly seems to be making probability statements about the unknown parameter. If we see the statement that [3.5, 11.6] is a 95% confidence interval for a parameter $\mu$, is this saying that there is a 95% chance that $\mu$ lies between 3.5 and 11.6? No, it is instead saying that if we repeated this experiment a great many times and calculated an interval each time according to the rule used to get the interval [3.5, 11.6], then 95% of those intervals would contain $\mu$. The 95% probability is a property of the rule that was used to create the interval, not of the interval itself. It is simply not allowed, and would be wrong, to attribute that probability to the actual interval [3.5, 11.6]. This is a very unintuitive argument, and frequentist statements such as these are widely misinterpreted, even by trained statisticians. The erroneous interpretation of the confidence interval—that there is a 95% chance of the parameter $\mu$ lying in the particular interval [3.5, 11.6]—is almost universally made by statistician and nonstatistician alike.

In a Bayesian analysis, the parameters do have probability distributions, and if a Bayesian analysis produces a 95% interval, then it does have exactly the interpretation that is usually put on a confidence interval. The fact that practitioners invariably wish to interpret a confidence interval in this way is evidence that the Bayesian approach is more natural and gives more direct answers to the practitioners' questions. An entirely similar argument can be made about frequentist significance tests. If a null hypothesis is rejected with a p-value of 1% in a study (call this sample A), this does not mean that this hypothesis has only a 1% probability of being true. Instead, it means that if we took a great many samples from a single population and calculated the test statistics, less than 1% of all the possible test statistics would assume a value greater than the one obtained in sample A. Note that this statement has no probabilistic claims about the hypothesis itself. To interpret a *p*-value in this way is not only wrong but dangerously wrong. Only a Bayesian analysis can (and does) give a probability that a hypothesis is true or false.

Underlying this distinction between the two approaches to statistics is a difference in how they interpret probability itself. In frequentist statistics, a probability can only be a long-run limiting relative frequency. This is the familiar definition used in elementary courses, often motivated by ideas like tossing coins a very large number of times and looking at the long-run limiting frequency of "heads." Bayesian statistics, in contrast, rest on an interpretation of probability as a personal degree of belief. Although this seems woolly and unscientific, it is important to recognize that Bayesian statisticians have developed analyses based on this interpretation very widely and successfully. The necessity of such an interpretation becomes clearer when we appreciate how many events that we would be willing to consider as having probabilities could never have a frequentist probability. The probability of a hypothesis is an obvious example, since a particular hypothesis either is or is not true, and we cannot consider any experimental repetitions of it as we could for tossing a coin. The probability of rain tomorrow is another example: Tomorrow is a unique day, with meteorological conditions preceding it today that have not existed in precisely the same form before and never will again. Most of the uncertain events and variables of real interest to scientists and practitioners are one-off things, and a Bayesian approach is necessary to accommodate our wish to describe them by probabilities.

This distinction leads us to the second major difference in practice between Bayesian and frequentist analysis. When a Bayesian analysis reports a probability interval for a parameter, this is a **posterior interval**, derived from the parameter's **posterior distribution**, based not only on the data but also on whatever other information or knowledge the investigator has. Before seeing the data, the investigator has a **prior distribution**, based only on that other information, known as prior information. The Bayesian approach combines the prior distribution with the information in the data to obtain the posterior distribution, from which any inferences are derived. The mathematical tool for combining these two sources of information is Bayes' theorem, which is why the approach is called "Bayesian."

## Value and Use

In general, the power of Bayesian methods derives from

- Their more natural inference statements, which address the real questions of interest (as in giving a posterior probability of a hypothesis being true, instead of a *p*-value that seems to say the same but whose real interpretation is much more convoluted);
- Their relevance to the decision-making process, as they allow probabilistic statements about the parameter values or future outcomes;
- Their ability to incorporate other, often more judgmental, sources of information than the immediate data (in the form of a prior distribution); and
- Their framework to estimate value of information;

These are of as much value in health economics as elsewhere. An example of a parameter is the incremental cost-effectiveness ratio for treatment A over treatment B. The ratio is not repeatable and cannot be the subject of frequentist probability statements. In a Bayesian analysis, we can formally state the probability that the ratio lies below some threshold, whereas this is *not* what a frequentist *p*-value gives us.

Wherever statistical methods are used in health economics, it is possible to apply a Bayesian approach.

One area where the use of Bayesian methods is already widespread without being recognized is in probabilistic sensitivity analysis of economic models. Sensitivity analysis (*see term:* Sensitivity Analysis) attempts to quantify the consequences on outputs of the model as a result of uncertainty about the inputs (since input parameters for such models are frequently known only imperfectly). The probabilistic technique for sensitivity analysis puts probability distributions on the inputs (and computes the implied probability distribution of relevant outputs, usually by simulation). The point is that these distributions in practice only can be Bayesian, representing degrees of belief about those parameters, since they cannot have a frequentist interpretation.

## Issues

A key issue in any use of Bayesian analysis is the origin and nature of the prior distribution. The use of the investigator's own prior information and beliefs is a potentially contentious issue, and this is the main reason why Bayesian methods have been viewed with suspicion. This is even more true for Bayesian analysis in health economics, because of the natural insistence by regulatory agencies on objective appraisal of the evidence. Responses to this demand for objectivity include the use of prior distributions that try to be objectively noninformative and so allow the data alone to influence the conclusions. However, this may fail to make use of valuable information, and future uses of Bayesian methods in health economics are likely to seek to clarify the kinds of information that will be acceptable. It is worth noting that the Food and Drug Administration in the United States has formally approved the use of Bayesian methods in submissions on medical devices. In the United Kingdom, the National Institute of Clinical Excellence (NICE) has acknowledged, at least in principle, that Bayesian methods may be used to support cost-effectiveness claims.

Another issue is that Bayesian methods are typically more complex and require more substantial computing resources than frequentist methods. This is compounded by the fact that standard software packages do not yet incorporate Bayesian analyses.

## BIBLIOGRAPHY

Briggs AH. A Bayesian approach to stochastic cost-effectiveness analysis. *Health Econ.* 1999;8: 257–261.

Jones DA. A Bayesian approach to the economic evaluation of health care technologies. In: B Spilker, ed. *Quality of Life and Pharmacoeconomics in Clinical Trials.* 2nd ed. Philadelphia: Lippincott-Raven; 1996.

O'Hagan A, Stevens JW, Montmartin J. Inference for the C/E acceptability curve and C/E ratio. *Pharmacoeconomics.* 2000;17:339–349.

# Biotechnology
## Biopharmaceutical
## Biological Drug
## Vaccines
## Gene Therapy

## BRIEF DEFINITION

**Biotechnology** is the manipulation of living organisms or their components to solve problems or to make useful products. It is a collection of technologies that capitalize on the attributes of cells and biological molecules, such as DNA and proteins. Biotechnology contributes to such diverse areas as human health and medicine, food production, criminal investigations, and waste management.

## EXPLANATION

Although biotechnology has been around for centuries, recent developments in DNA technology have launched a revolution in the field. Early examples of biotechnology may be traced to 5000 B.C. when diverse strains of plants or animals were selectively bred to produce greater genetic variation and more desirable traits. For example, corn (maize) was one of the first food crops known to have been cultivated by human beings, yet no wild forms of the plant have been found, indicating that corn was most likely the result of some early agricultural experiments. Another common biotechnology practice that goes back centuries is the use of microbes to make wine and cheese. These early examples of biotechnology relied on natural genetic processes, such as mutation and genetic recombination.

The modern era of biotechnology began in 1953 when James Watson and Francis Crick presented their double helix model of DNA. Several other significant advances in technology followed, such as Werner Arber's discovery in the 1960s of restriction enzymes in bacteria and Stanley Cohen and Herbert Boyer's use of restriction enzymes to insert a specific gene from one bacterium into another bacterium. Soon scientists were able to transfer genes from other animals, including humans, into bacteria. These transgenic bacteria, bacteria to which a gene from another species has been transferred, were able to produce a product, such as human growth hormone or human insulin, for which the bacteria had no use but which would greatly benefit mankind. These advances marked the beginning of recombinant DNA technology (genetic engineering), an example of modern biotechnology based on the manipulation of DNA in vitro. This technology now allows scientists to modify specific genes and move them between organisms as distinct as bacteria, plants, and animals.

A **biopharmaceutical** refers to a pharmaceutical product manufactured by biotechnology methods or processes, generally involving live biological organisms or components. In contrast to a conventional drug with a known structure that are chemically synthesized, a biopharmaceutical is derived from living organisms and may contain complex mixtures that are not easily identified or characterized. Biopharmaceuticals include microorganisms, animal cell and tissue-derived proteins, vaccines, blood products, antibodies, enzymes, cytokines, radio-immune conjugates, and certain engineered tissue grafts or implants. A biotechnology product may be considered biopharmaceutical whether it is derived using old (e.g., fermentation) or new (e.g., recombinant DNA, monoclonal antibody) methods.

The US Food and Drug Administration (FDA) categorizes a **biological drug** as biopharmaceutical. Biological drugs include any virus, therapeutic serum, toxin, antitoxin, vaccine, blood, blood component or derivative, allergenic product, or analogous product that is applicable to the prevention, treatment, or cure of diseases or injuries to humans. Some examples include, but are not limited to, bacterial and viral vaccines, human blood and plasma and their derivatives, and certain products produced through biotechnology such as interferons and erythropoietins.

### VALUE AND USE

Biotechnology medicines and therapies use proteins, antibodies, and other substances naturally produced in the human body to fight infections and disease. In addition, other living organisms, such as viruses, bacteria, yeasts, and plant and animal cells are used to assist in the large-scale production of medicines for human use. More than 250 million people worldwide have been helped by the biotechnology drug products and vaccines approved by the FDA. Of the biotech medicines on the market, more than 75 percent were approved in the last six years, and there are hundreds more products and vaccines currently in clinical trials.

There are four primary areas of health care which rely on biotechnology:

1. *Medicines.* The primary medicines approved today are proteins that help the body fight infections or carry out specific functions. The FDA has approved medicines to treat anemia, cystic fibrosis, growth deficiency, hemophilia, leukemia, hepatitis, genital warts, transplant rejection, and some forms of cancer.

2. *Vaccines.* Vaccines help the body recognize and fight disease. Conventional vaccines use weakened or killed forms of a virus or bacteria to introduce antigens to the body that the immune system uses to identify the pathogen. The body then produces antibodies that help to build a resistance to the disease. A biotechnology vaccine consists of only the antigen, not the actual microbe, thus eliminating the risk of transmitting the actual virus or bacterium. The FDA has approved the use of a biotech vaccine for hepatitis B and research is being conducted for other vaccines to combat influenza, AIDS, herpes viruses, cholera, Rocky Mountain spotted fever, and several diarrheal diseases.

3. *Diagnostics.* Biotechnology diagnostics may be used to detect a wide variety of diseases and genetic conditions. Some examples are diagnostic tests to screen donated blood from HIV and hepatitis, low-density lipoprotein ("bad" cholesterol) blood tests, and home pregnancy tests.

4. *Gene therapy* (*see term:* Gene Therapy). Gene therapy uses the genes themselves as drugs to treat hereditary genetic disorders by replacing a faulty or missing gene. Gene therapy has been used to treat severe combined immunodeficiency disease and to introduce new cells to produce cell-growth factor or to perform a beneficial cellular function.

In addition to the health care industry, biotechnology has made a dramatic impact on the world in other areas. Consumers are already enjoying many biotechnology foods such as papaya, soybeans, and corn. In addition, hundreds of biopesticides and other agricultural products are being used to improve our food supply and reduce our dependence on conventional chemical pesticides. Using pollution-eating microbes, environmental biotechnology products have advanced waste management and have helped develop more efficient ways to clean up hazardous waste. Industrial biotechnology applications have led to cleaner processes that produce less waste and use less energy and water than past production methods for such products as paper, textiles, and detergents. DNA fingerprinting has dramatically improved criminal investigations and forensic medicine, and the technology has led to significant advances in anthropology and wildlife management. Even the mining industry has found application for biotechnology, such as the use of bacteria to help purify low-grade ores of copper. The advances made through biotechnology are simply too numerous to count.

ISSUES

Some people, including many scientists, object to any procedure that changes the genetic composition of an organism. They are concerned that genetically altered organisms may eliminate existing species or otherwise upset the natural balance of living things. Some are also concerned that biotechnology may inadvertently produce extremely virulent pathogenic microorganisms that if accidentally released into the environment will cause worldwide epidemics. Other critics of biotechnology are concerned with the ethical dilemmas associated with the production of transgenic organisms. Since biopharmaceuticals typically require extensive purification techniques, there are concerns about communicable diseases increasing as an indirect result of these purification processes and even the sometimes-vague characterization of these new drugs. There are also concerns about less developed nations with extremely limited financial resources: are biotechnology methods sustainable in these countries without continuous outside technical and material support? Finally, there are numerous concerns about biotechnology being used to produce biological weapons of mass destruction.

BIBLIOGRAPHY

Behizad M, Curling JM. Comparing the safety of synthetic and biological ligands used for the purification of therapeutic proteins. *Biopharm.* 2000;13:42–46.
Huete-Perez JA, Orozco DA. Biotech gap between north and south. *Science.* 2001;294:2289–2290.
Singer PA, Daar AS. Harnessing genomics and biotechnology to improve global health equity. *Science.* 2001;294:87–89.

# Bootstrapping

BRIEF DEFINITION

**Bootstrapping** is a technique to approximate the accuracy (e.g., confidence interval or standard error) of a statistical estimate.

EXPLANATION

The nonparametric bootstrap is a useful general device for approximating the true distribution of a computed estimate (e.g., sample mean) without making assumptions about the distribution underlying the original data. It is based on the idea of drawing many "bootstrap" samples from the original data. A single bootstrap sample is a sample of the same size, n, as the original sample, and drawn from that original sample with replacement (i.e., the same member of the original sample can be drawn more than once). For instance, if the original sample comprises n = 10 values 1, 2, 4, 5, 7, 8, 9, 12, 14, 20, then a bootstrap sample might comprise 2, 4, 4, 8, 8, 8, 9, 12, 20, 20.

Bootstrapping entails drawing a large number of bootstrap samples, say N = 1000 or more. From each bootstrap sample, we calculate a value for the desired measure T. After N samples, we have N sampled values for T. These N values can be used to approximate the true distribution of T, no matter what the underlying distribution of the original data might have been. Likewise, the standard deviation of these N sampled T's approximates the true standard error of T. The interval spanning the central 95% of these T's is an approximate 95% confidence interval for true T.

There are many variations on this simple description of the bootstrap. In particular, there are several different ways to construct a confidence interval from the bootstrap sample of T values.

The larger the size, n, of the original sample, the better the approximation produced through bootstrapping. Notice that the quality of the approximation does not depend on the number (N) of bootstrap samples we draw. The number of samples drawn needs to be large, but only in order to calculate the bootstrap inferences accurately. Drawing a very large number of samples means that we calculate a bootstrap confidence interval more accurately, but what we have calculated is still only approximately valid as a confidence interval.

## VALUE AND USE

Bootstrapping is widely advocated in health economics, particularly because of the skewed nature of the distributions of costs. It is clearly unrealistic to assume that cost distributions are normal, and we may be unwilling to assume any other specific distributional form. Therefore, bootstrapping is used to make inferences about parameters like mean cost and incremental ratio.

Bootstrapping is used particularly for incremental cost-effectiveness ratios because alternative methods for ratios are especially problematic.

## ISSUES

An alternative nonparametric method is based on the central limit theorem, which says that the means of samples are approximately normally distributed, no matter what the distribution of the individual data items. This is also attractive in the context of health economics since it is in general the mean cost and effectiveness (and other measures computed from them, like the incremental cost-effectiveness ratio or incremental net benefit) that are of interest. Like the bootstrap theory, the central limit theorem says that the quality of the approximation (that sample means have normal distributions) improves with the size of the original sample.

It is not clear in practice whether the bootstrap or the central limit theorem will give a better approximation in any given situation, and neither may be good if the sample size is small. If used, for example, in a large trial yielding data on many hundreds of patients, then the bootstrap should be reliable. With a sample size of 30 or fewer, it is doubtful whether the bootstrap should be used.

## BIBLIOGRAPHY

Briggs AH, Wonderling DE, Mooney CZ. Pulling cost-effectiveness analysis up by its bootstraps: A non-parametric approach to confidence interval estimation. *Health Econ.* 1997;6:327–340.

Efron B, Tibshirani RJ. *An Introduction to the Bootstrap.* New York: Chapman and Hall; 1993.

O'Hagan A, Stevens JW (2003). Assessing and comparing costs: how robust are the bootstrap and methods based on asymptotic normality? *Health Econ.* 2003;12:33–49.

# Case Mix Index
Case Mix
Risk Adjustment
Severity Adjustment

## BRIEF DEFINITION
The **case mix index** (CMI) is one measure or indicator of the average relative weight of diagnosis-related groups (DRGs) assigned to hospitalized patients treated at the same institution.

## EXPLANATION
After Medicare's prospective payment system (PPS) went into effect in the early 1980s, the case mix index was developed to monitor hospital charges. The Prospective Payment Assessment Commission (ProPAC) is one agency that tracks CMI to monitor trends in hospital charges. Higher CMIs equate to higher aggregate hospital charges for the DRG mix of patients being treated at a given hospital. Thus, if hospital A is treating a higher number of patients with multiple health conditions or more serious health conditions than hospital B, then the CMI will capture this assuming higher charges are seen in hospital A. The term **case mix** is often confused with the terms **risk adjustment** and **severity adjustment**. What differentiates these two terms from case mix index is the fact that they predict an outcome using risk factors and modeling techniques. In contrast, the Medicare case mix index is based solely on past trends of hospital charges for the mix of patients treated at the hospital. The goal of CMI is to forecast variation of resource utilization for entire populations based on past trends at the hospital level. Thus facilities are compared to other facilities using CMI.

DRGs are a classification system that groups patients according to diagnosis, type of treatment, age, and other relevant criteria. Under the prospective payment system, hospitals are paid a set fee for treating patients in a single DRG category, regardless of the actual cost of care for any individual.

## VALUE AND USE
Case mix index is used to monitor and set the payment systems to hospitals. Medicare payments to hospitals are directly tied to the CMI. For every one-percentage point in CMI, hospitals are paid millions of dollars more in government payments. Although the system was originally designed by Medicare, other payers may also use the CMI to monitor trends in the patients being seen

at hospitals and to compare hospitals using the CMI. In this manner, the payers can use the CMI to assess resource use within a given population. Then the payers can more accurately and efficiently plan and use resources. Currently, efforts are under way to develop case mix indexes appropriate for outpatient settings. However, these appear to be in the beginning stages of development at this time.

### Issues

One significant issue related to CMI is the idea of DRG "creep"—the idea that coding of patients' primary and secondary discharge may change to upgrade a hospital's CMI. Studies have found this to occur. In fact, ever since the PPS was implemented, the average CMI has increased every year. Changing coding practices causes some of this effect. However, some of the effect is caused by the use of new technology, the aging of the US population, increased use of health care services, etc. It is very difficult to separate the effects on CMI of coding and these other factors. The practice of linking discharge codes (ICD-9-CM) to hospital payment has always been questioned from a clinical credibility point of view.

### Bibliography

Carter GM, Newhouse JP, Relles DA. *How Much Change in the Case Mix Index Is DRG Creep?* Santa Monica, Calif: Rand Corporation; 1990.

Iezzoni LI. *Risk Adjustment for Measuring Health Care Outcomes.* Ann Arbor, Mich: Healthcare Administration Press, 1997.

Weiner JP, Starfield BH, Steinwachs DM, et al. Development and application of a population-oriented measure of ambulatory care case mix. *Med Care.* 1991;29:453–472.

# Clinical Practice Guidelines

### Brief Definition

**Clinical practice guidelines** (CPGs) are user-friendly, evidence-based, systematically developed statements that assist primary health care providers and patients in making appropriate decisions for specific clinical circumstances.

### Explanation

Guidelines regarding appropriate care existed in ancient times, but now the emphasis is placed on systematically developed and evidence-based guidelines. In the past, CPGs focused on quality-enhancing guidelines, whereas current CPG development results from outcomes research focusing on effectiveness and cost-justifiability of diagnostic and therapeutic procedures. Established standards, such as evidence-based medicine, are implemented to ensure scientific validity and clarity of communication of CPGs.
Good CPGs

- Define questions occurring in the practice and explicitly identify all decision options and outcomes;

- Identify, appraise, and summarize best given evidence regarding prevention, diagnosis, prognosis, therapy, harm, and cost-effectiveness in a manner most relevant to decision makers; and

- Explicitly identify decision points at which integration of valid evidence and clinical experience should help with making the best decision for the patient.

Key components of a useful CPG include

- Identification of the key decisions and their consequences;
- Review of the relevant, valid evidence on the benefits, risks, and costs of alternative decisions; and
- Presentation of the evidence required to inform key decisions in a simple, accessible format that is flexible.

The following attributes of CPGs are considered desirable:

- Validity—strength of evidence and estimated outcome
- Reliability/reproducibility
- Clinical applicability
- Clinical flexibility
- Clarity
- Multidisciplinary process
- Scheduled review
- Comprehensive documentation and description

Unfortunately it is not always possible to maintain all of the above-mentioned attributes in every single CPG, and guideline developers are confronted with numerous hurdles.

Information from medical literature is systematically obtained and critically appraised with evidence-based methods. Evidence-based guidelines, however, are limited insofar as cost is most often not considered. A global subjective agreement of experts (consensus method) is the most commonly used method of guideline development in New Zealand. Unfortunately the biases of the experts cannot be removed. Guideline developers may also request comprehensive and systematic overviews from groups such as the Cochrane Collaboration, the York Center for Reviews and Dissemination, and the United States Agency for Health Care Policy and Research.

### VALUE AND USE

Practice guidelines are not fixed protocols that have to be followed; rather, they should be considered and applied with professional judgment. They should never substitute for clinical judgment but should play an assisting role only. They are meant to guide physicians toward delivering high-quality care in a cost-effective manner. Deviations from given CPGs might be necessary depending on the patient's individual circumstances and needs.

Practice guidelines are available for all kinds of diseases and interventions.

Internet Web sites also provide information on evidence-based CPGs to health care professionals, usually for expert audiences in the health care sector and health professionals.

## ISSUES

The use and credibility of CPGs are still debated among physicians. A CPG developed according to the principles of epidemiology, which deals with large patient populations, is often not applicable to the individual patient's needs. Evidence-based practice and evidence-based clinical guidelines should be valid for the individual patient, but presented as formal overviews they are not in a form directly relevant to individual patient care. Guidelines will be more useful for real-life clinical decision making if they present evidence applicable to the individual patient. On the other hand, CPGs that maximize benefits for individual patients do not necessarily maximize cost-effectiveness for populations of patients, which complicates the situation even further as financial resources become even scarcer. In cost-effectiveness studies, mathematical techniques, collectively known as optimization, may be implemented to maximize or minimize key variables for investigating clinical options, which benefits the population and individual patient successively. Furthermore, guidelines produced by various organizations, for the same intervention, may differ. Therefore rigorous criteria have been developed to combat this lack of uniformity in design, structure, and presentation of CPGs.

CPGs could influence physician behavior; however, they always allow for the physician to exercise his or her own judgment. Practice guidelines should improve the quality and appropriateness of care as well as contain the cost of health care. In the United States, in some states, a physician who acts in compliance with CPGs may use this as an affirmative defense in court.

Of course each patient is unique; but taking a standard approach to the patient's condition can result in optimal medical care, reduction in legal risks, and lower health care costs.

## BIBLIOGRAPHY

Eddy DM. *Clinical Decision Making.* Sudbury, Mass: Jones and Bartlett Publishers; 1996.

Field M, Lohr K, eds. *Guidelines for Clinical Practice: From Development to Use.* Washington, DC: National Academy Press; 1992.

Granata AV, Hillman AL. Competing practice guidelines: using cost-effectiveness analysis to make optimal decisions. *Ann Intern Med.* 1998;128:56–63.

# Clinical Trial

Randomized Clinical Trial
Mega-Trial
Firms Trial
Head-to-Head Comparison Study
Equivalence Study
Nonrandomized Trial with
    Contemporaneous Controls
Nonrandomized Trial with
    Historical Controls
Case-Control Study
Cross-Sectional Study
Case Report Study
Crossover Trial

Open-Label Trial
Double-Blind Study
Single-Blind Study
Matched-Pair Study
Clinical Endpoint
Clinical Indicator
Economic Clinical Trial
Piggyback Study
Bridging Study
Clinical Research Study
Prospective Clinical Research Study
Retrospective Clinical Research Study

## BRIEF DEFINITION

A **clinical trial** is a research study to test the safety, efficacy, and/or effectiveness of a health care intervention (such as a new protocol and treatment) intended to alleviate a specific disease condition in human subjects; it is a prospective experimental study comparing the effect and value of preventive, diagnostic, or therapeutic intervention(s) in human beings under control conditions. In such a trial, there are at least two groups being compared: intervention and control. Controls receive either placebo or existing therapy. When a clinical trial is controlled, the assignment of subjects to the treatment groups should be randomized. Clinical trials of experimental drugs typically proceed through four phases, known as Phase I, Phase II, Phase III, and Phase IV clinical trials. While these phases are performed sequentially, they may overlap. Regulatory approval is typically granted upon successful completion of Phase III trials.

New therapies are only tested in humans after promising and thorough animal and laboratory research studies have been conducted.

Clinical trial phases are described as follows:

*Phase I* clinical trials are the initial assessment of a product in humans. Their purpose is to establish the product's safety, safe dose range, and pharmacokinetic properties. Safety is judged by side effects or toxicities that occur. Pharmacokinetic properties are typically measured by determining the product's absorption, distribution, metabolism, and elimination within the body. A typical Phase I study involves 20 to 80 healthy volunteers who do not have the disease being studied.

*Phase II* clinical trials build upon the information obtained in Phase I studies. The purpose of Phase II studies is to evaluate safety and efficacy and determine the most appropriate dose for the treatment. Phase II clinical trials are usually performed on 100 to 300 or more subjects who have the disease or condition of interest. Subjects selected to participate have the condition of interest and may have comorbidities.

*Phase III* clinical trials confirm the efficacy of an experimental drug and further establish its safety profile in a much larger patient population. Phase III trials are typically conducted on several thousand people with the disease, where possible, to establish more definitively the safety and efficacy of the treatment agent at various doses. The drug is often given for much longer periods of time (sometimes two to four years) to subjects with the condition of interest, who frequently have other health problems as well, to replicate the patient population in the "real" world. These trials provide data required for regulatory approval and form the basis for how the product should be prescribed. Phase III clinical trials are typically controlled compared to either existing treatment or placebo. It is estimated that only one in every five products that enter Phase I studies makes it through the completion of Phase III studies.

*Phase IV* clinical trials are conducted after a product has been approved and are frequently known as postmarketing studies. These studies continue testing the drug or treatment to collect information about its effect in various populations and any side effects associated with long-term use. In Phase IV clinical trials, the postapproval monitoring and analysis of the treatment agent is conducted as the agent is used in the general population of diseased patients, rather than in the carefully controlled and restricted population of the earlier phase clinical trials. In essence, Phase IV trials assess the actual effectiveness and sometimes also costs and patient-reported outcomes of the treatment.

## EXPLANATION AND VALUE AND USE

Results of clinical trials play an important role in pharmacoeconomics. The economic value of a particular health care intervention depends in part, if not mostly or entirely, on the intervention's clinical value. That value, in terms of efficacy, effectiveness, and safety, is typically measured in clinical trials. Increasingly, the value of an intervention in terms of economic outcomes and patient-reported outcomes is also being assessed in clinical trials. Several types of clinical trial designs exist and are briefly described below. Prior to those descriptions, several terms important to the design and conduct of these studies are described.

In pure observational studies of practice and associated outcomes, it is difficult to ascribe causality to observed relationships between treatment and outcomes because numerous patient, provider, and environmental factors may confound those relationships. Accordingly, in a clinical trial, to reduce if not eliminate these sources of bias, subjects are typically assigned to a specific study arm on the basis of randomization, which is the assignment of subjects to alternative interventions by using a probabilistic rule such that neither the investigator nor the patient can predict the intervention assigned at the moment of inclusion.

A well-designed clinical trial protocol is essential to ensure the quality and integrity of a trial. The protocol is a plan that states the study objectives and describes the design and methodology: how the clinical trial is to be carried out and how the data are to be collected and analyzed. Study objectives are concise and precise statements of prespecified hypotheses. The target population to which the study results are inferred is characterized through specific inclusion and exclusion criteria. The design should also include a baseline assessment of relevant data to be done after each subject's informed consent is obtained and before the subject receives any intervention. A description of the interventions to be compared and the specific study design (parallel, crossover, etc) is fundamental.

One of the most important decisions is the definition of the control group whose outcomes are being contrasted with those of subjects receiving the alternative intervention(s). Clinical trials are frequently conducted with active control agents to establish the superiority of the new intervention versus the standard treatment. If an effective and safe alternative therapy does not exist, a placebo control group—a group receiving a drug or procedure with no intrinsic therapeutic value—is used to provide an unbiased assessment of the effectiveness and safety of the therapy under study. An important aspect to prevent bias caused by subjective judgments in reporting, evaluation, data processing, and statistical analysis is the use of blinding—an experimental condition in which various groups involved in the trial are withheld from the knowledge of the treatments assigned to patients.

Finally, to assess the efficacy of the intervention under study, in any clinical trial it is necessary to determine the endpoints, the quantitative measurements implied or required by the objectives. Although clinical endpoints—traditional medical measures of a therapy's impact, such as serum cholesterol levels, metabolic rate, tumor size, absence of infection, or survival time—are frequently used, other endpoints more related to the patient's perception of therapy results, such as patient satisfaction or quality of life (patient-reported outcomes), are being used increasingly as are economic endpoints. In any case, the method of endpoint assessment must be prespecified, accurate, and free of bias.

Regulatory agencies use clinical trials to understand the safety and efficacy of an intervention (pharmaceutical, biotechnologic, or device), so that appropriate registration decisions can be made. Ideally only interventions shown to be safe and efficacious will be made and remain available to their populations. Clinical trials are designed to answer the question: "Does this intervention do what it is supposed to do, and is it safe in doing that proposed use?" Types of studies include the following.

A **randomized clinical trial** tests the safety and efficacy of a health care intervention by randomly recruiting participants into either the treatment or the control group. Random refers to the placement of participants into a study arm based solely on chance and not on the preferences or influence of the physician, patient, or trial sponsors. Random assignment is useful because it allows one to assume that all treatment arms contain subjects with roughly equivalent characteristics and that the measured outcomes are due to the intervention and not to differences in subject characteristics.

A **mega-trial** is a massive randomized clinical trial that tests the outcomes of drugs or other health care interventions by enrolling 10000 or more subjects. Mega-trials enable sponsors to evaluate outcomes that are relatively rare. Typically these studies involve numerous study sites, sometimes in multiple countries and continents.

A **firms trial** is a randomized clinical trial in which subjects are randomized among entire clinics or other institutional settings. In the firms trial, subjects are randomized to control clinics versus treatment clinics as opposed to control or treatment groups within a single clinic.

A **head-to-head comparison study** is a randomized clinical trial where two health care interventions known to have the desired outcome are compared to determine which intervention is more efficacious for the desired outcome.

An **equivalence study** is designed to evaluate whether the outcomes of a health care intervention are clinically equal to those of the alternative technology. The measures that these types of studies require are different from those required in trials trying to demonstrate a difference. In addition, measures will vary greatly depending on whether the comparison is an attempt to show equivalent health outcomes between two different substances or an attempt to show bioequivalence and therapeutic interchangeability between two versions of a similar substance. The latter is a very complex process for which guidelines are still being established.

A **nonrandomized trial with contemporaneous controls** is a trial in which the treatment group is compared with a "similar" cohort receiving care in the same setting by the same providers but not receiving the treatment within the same time frame. A "similar" cohort is established by matching patients based on a set of demographic and clinical characteristics (e.g., age, sex, duration of disease, concomitant diagnoses) that may have an impact on the outcome being measured.

A **nonrandomized trial with historical controls** is a comparison of the cohort receiving the intervention with a "similar" cohort that received care (but not the intervention being evaluated) in the same setting by the same providers, during another time period (usually earlier).

A **case-control study** is an observational epidemiological study that starts with the identification of a group of individuals (cases) with the disease of interest, and a group of individuals (controls) without the disease who are otherwise similar to the cases. It is a retrospective or prospective study in which participants are selected on the basis of presence or absence of an event or condition of interest. The relationship of a risk factor (e.g., exposure to a physical agent, receipt of a screening test) to the disease is evaluated by determining how frequently the risk factor is present in cases and controls.

A **cross-sectional study** examines the relationship between diseases and other variables of interest as they exist in a defined population at one particular time. It is an evaluation based on a single snapshot in time, and no longitudinal (follow-up) data are available.

A **case report study** is an analysis that profiles a single patient and describes the treatment pattern and outcomes.

A **crossover trial** is a study in which each subject receives both treatments being compared, or the treatment and placebo, in two consecutive time periods, or in two periods separated by a washout period. Such trials are used for patients who have a stable, usually chronic, condition during both treatment periods. Each participant serves as his or her own control. In a crossover trial, within-patient differences, or variability in outcomes within each patient, are used to assess treatment value.

An **open-label trial** is a study in which both subjects and investigators know which product the subject is receiving. This is in contrast to a **double-blind study**, in which neither subject nor researcher knows this information, or a **single-blind study** where only one party (typically the physician and not the subject) knows.

A **matched-pair study** is a type of parallel trial design in which investigators identify pairs of subjects who are "identical" with respect to relevant factors, then randomize them so that one receives Treatment A and the other Treatment B.

A **clinical endpoint** is a consequence of the use of health care products, services, or programs that affect a patient's clinical well-being. Usually it is a medical measure of an intervention's impact on the body, such as serum cholesterol levels, metabolic rate, tumor size, or absence of infection. Clinical endpoints may be either intermediate ("surrogate") endpoints or final endpoints.

A **clinical indicator** is an agreed-upon measure, process, or outcome used to judge a particular clinical situation and indicate whether the care delivered was appropriate. Examples include whether antibiotics were administered before surgery and the rate of adverse reactions in response to the antibiotics.

An **economic clinical trial** is a study in which the objectives and methodology are specifically designed to provide analysis or assessment of the resource use and cost implications as well as the clinical effectiveness of the intervention.

A **piggyback study** is an economic study (involving economic data collection and analysis components) that is added onto and therefore a part of a clinical trial originally focused on clinical issues.

A **bridging study** determines the safety and tolerance of a drug in a target population and aids in the selection of appropriate doses for subsequent efficacy studies.

A **clinical research study** may have either a prospective or retrospective design. **Prospective clinical research study** involves the collection of data on clinical endpoints, treatments, and related measures forward in time. A **retrospective clinical research study** involves the analysis of clinical outcomes that is already present in existing databases.

Because a prospective clinical study is designed to meet certain objectives by collecting new data, it can be designed to enable the collection of more detailed clinical and related information from patients over time. In contrast, a retrospective clinical study uses existing patient data, generally created for different purposes (e.g., administrative databases of medical claims). Both prospective and retrospective clinical studies are designed to contribute to knowledge about clinical outcomes associated with existing therapies in naturalistic, "real-world" settings.

## ISSUES

Every clinical study design has advantages and disadvantages. As a result, the design and methods of studies must be examined along with the findings to understand the clinical literature in any particular therapeutic area.

Randomized, controlled clinical trials offer internal validity and reasonable confidence that the treatment effects observed in the study reflect true treatment effects. However, if the study sample is not representative of the population or the care of patients in the study does not accurately reflect true real-world care, the external validity of the trial results is questionable.

This is typically framed as an issue of efficacy versus effectiveness. Randomized clinical trials offer data on the efficacy, costs, and/or other outcomes of an intervention in a controlled setting. Health economic analyses are concerned with the effectiveness of the intervention in the real world, certainly an "uncontrolled" setting and one that is often difficult to understand given only randomized clinical trial data. Differences between efficacy as assessed in controlled trials and effectiveness in real practice may be attributable to such factors as access to care, cost, compliance and persistence, and other patient, provider, or societal factors not typically addressed in randomized controlled trials.

Increasingly, sponsors of clinical trials understand the importance of assessing economic value and patient-reported outcomes within these studies along with the clinical outcomes. However, one must be careful to describe carefully the primary and secondary objectives of a trial. Although analysis and ascertainment of primary objectives may be attainable with a particular protocol, the same study characteristics that make that possible may hinder the ascertainment of the secondary objectives. More often than not, understanding of economic and patient-reported outcomes is characterized as a secondary objective. As a result, the true ability of a clinical trial to measure these aspects of the value of a health care intervention may be suboptimal, and as a result, other research may be necessary.

## BIBLIOGRAPHY

Benson K, Hartz AJ. A comparison of observational studies and randomized, controlled trials. *N Engl J Med.* 2000;342:1878–1886.

CDER Learn. http://www.fda.gov/cder/learn/CDERLearn/default.htm. Accessed March 31, 2003.

Concato J, Shah N, Horwitz RI. Randomized, controlled trials, observational studies, and the hierarchy of research designs. *N Engl J Med.* 2000;342:1887–1892.

Greenberg R, Daniels S, Flanders D, et al. *Medical Epidemiology,* 2nd ed. Columbus, Ohio: Appleton and Lange; 1996.

Understanding Clinical Trials. http://clinicaltrials.gov. Accessed March 31, 2003.

# Clinical Trial – Study Bias

Study Bias
Selection Bias
Response Bias
Information Bias
Interviewer Bias
Site Selection Bias

## Brief Definition

**Study bias** is a systematic error in the design or conduct of a study that results in a distorted assessment of the intervention's impact on the outcome(s) measured. This undesirable characteristic can be introduced unwittingly into clinical studies by any characteristic or risk factor that systematically affects the results but is not due to the intervention being studied. As such, it is distinct from random error, which is error that occurs when sampling a subset of subjects from a much larger population.

## Explanation

Although the potential for study bias may be greater for observational studies, clinical trials are also susceptible to this undesired effect. Types of study bias include:

**Selection bias:** A type of bias that occurs when selected, eligible study subjects do not participate in the clinical trial. This type of bias can occur if certain eligible patients are not asked to participate (e.g., the clinician believes the patient will not respond to the treatment) or if the patient refuses to participate (for reasons that might be related to treatment outcomes). The tendency for clinical trials to have restrictive eligibility criteria (e.g., based on gender, age, clinical characteristics, concomitant medications) is sometimes thought to cause selection bias. However, these eligibility criteria affect the study's generalizability (also called representativeness or external validity) rather than causing selection bias per se.

**Response bias:** A type of bias caused by study subjects not participating in part or all of the study data collection. Response bias can be thought of as a type of selection bias. It is frequently associated with a situation in which some subjects do not complete a study questionnaire, and therefore it also is called nonresponse bias or participation bias. Response bias will exist if the reasons that subjects do not participate (or return or complete a questionnaire) are differentially related to one of the study groups, either comparison or treatment (e.g., if subjects benefiting or not benefiting from the treatment are less likely to respond to the survey). The same type of bias can exist if subjects answer some but not all of the questions in a questionnaire; this is known as item nonresponse bias.

**Information bias:** A type of bias caused by inaccurate assessment of the study measures (also called misclassification bias). In clinical trials the measures frequently relate to the study outcomes. However, systematic errors can also occur in the assessment of exposure or study treatment. Due to poor compliance, many subjects in the treatment group may not actually take a medication they are expected to take, causing a type of misclassification bias. If the study is not blinded, then the subject or clinician may report a more favorable decrease of symptoms or greater improvement of other clinical measures for those in the treated group than in the comparison group. This will cause a differential misclassification bias that will exaggerate the treatment effect. Information bias will still occur if the misclassification is unrelated to the study group or treatment effect. This type of nondifferential misclassification bias will, in general, tend to decrease the observed treatment effect (i.e., a bias toward the null hypothesis of no effect).

**Interviewer bias:** A type of bias caused by the way interviewers administer the questionnaire or by the way the subjects respond to interviewers. Interviewer bias is a type of information bias related to the interaction between an interviewer and a subject. If interviewers probe for more detail or ask questions of certain subjects in a different way, then an inaccurate assessment might be made of the treatment effect. Likewise, if the subjects' responses are affected by the characteristics of interviewers and if there are differences in interviewers between treatment groups (e.g., the treated group is interviewed by physicians and the comparison group is interviewed by nurses), an interviewer bias might occur.

**Site selection bias:** A type of bias caused by the sites that participate in the study not being representative of the sites that would eventually use the intervention being studied. As with (subject) selection bias, site selection bias is a challenge to external validity (i.e., whether the results are generalizable to the relevant population).

## VALUE AND USE

Study bias can undermine the validity of a study. Biased study results can impact clinical decision making and public health policy by distorting the true value (or lack thereof) of a treatment or intervention.

It may be hard to evaluate whether certain types of bias exist in a study, especially from reading a published report of the findings. For example, it may not be possible to determine whether a subject's responses were affected by the interviewer's characteristics (interviewer bias). There should be some indication, however, that some types of biases are present. For example, the investigator should know and report the percentage of eligible patients who agreed to participate in the study and who completed all parts of the study protocol (indicators of possible selection bias and response bias).

Study bias may affect results in either direction, either exaggerating or underestimating a real treatment effect. In some cases, it may be possible to make an informed estimate as to the likely direction of the bias. Study bias may be very difficult, if not impossible, to correct during the analysis stage of a study. This highlights the fact that it should be addressed at the design, protocol development, data collection, and study monitoring stages. It is critical to have standardized procedures in place for conducting the study, including training and monitoring programs to minimize information bias. Also, well-defined, objective, and reproducible study endpoints are required, especially if the study is not blinded (i.e., if the study staff is aware of treatment group assignments).

## ISSUES

Randomization (i.e., patients are assigned at random to treatment group) and blinding (i.e., study staff and/or patients are not aware of the treatment assignment) are two important methods used in clinical trials to reduce the potential for study bias. Also, well-trained study staff that is familiar with the special requirements of clinical studies (beyond clinical care) can help minimize information bias and interviewer bias.

However, randomized, placebo-controlled, double-blind clinical trials (the "gold standard" of study designs) may still contain the types of bias cited above. Only a small percentage of people (who are not randomly selected) participate in clinical trials. The reasons why a person refuses to participate or why an investigator does not approach a subject about participating may lead to selection bias. Evaluating whether selection bias exists in a given study is difficult to evaluate because there is seldom a full accounting of who is eligible, who is approached, and who refuses to participate in clinical trials and why.

Participation at the beginning of a study does not necessarily mean complete participation throughout the study. Issues related to compliance, missed study visits, study withdrawal, and losses to follow-up can create study bias. Every effort should be made by the study staff to minimize these types of losses. If the reason for a subject's lack of adherence to the study protocol is related to the treatment or outcome, then study bias can occur. In these cases, special attention needs to be paid to the proper analytic approach (e.g., an intention-to-treat analysis) to avoid or at least minimize a biased assessment of the treatment effect.

## BIBLIOGRAPHY

Collet J, Boivin J, Spitzer W. Bias and confounding in pharmacoepidemiology. In: Strom B, ed. *Pharmacoepidemiology.* 2nd ed. Chichester, UK: John Wiley and Sons; 1994.

Collins R, MacMahon S. Reliable assessment of the effect of treatment on mortality and major morbidity, I: clinical trials. *Lancet.* 2001;357:373–380.

Pocock S. *Clinical Trials: A Practical Approach.* Chichester, UK: John Wiley and Sons; 1983.

# Compliance

Adherence
Treatment Persistence
Electronic Monitoring
Pill Count Method
Prescription Refill Rate
Attendance

BRIEF DEFINITION

Patient **compliance** (**adherence**) refers to the consistency and accuracy with which a patient follows a recommended medical regimen, usually referring to a pharmacotherapeutic regimen.

**Treatment persistence** refers to the continued use of the prescribed pharmacotherapeutic regimen or other program.

**Electronic monitoring** method is a measurement of the frequency and timing of doses taken by the patient compared to the frequency or timing that should occur based on the physician's prescription. Measurement is made by microprocessor driven devices that record the date and time of events. Data are transformed into patients' logs by special software.

**Pill count method** is a measurement of the amount of a drug remaining unused in the patient's possession compared to the amount that should be left based on the physician's prescription. This method is less accurate than electronic monitoring because patients often forget to return all of a medication.

**Prescription refill rate** refers to the measurement of the frequency or timing of prescription refills compared to the frequency or timing that should occur based on the physician's prescription. This method is less accurate than electronic monitoring because patients may obtain prescription refills without taking the medication.

**Attendance** refers to the measurement of the frequency or timing of medical follow-up visits compared to the frequency or timing that should occur based on the physician's plan.

Compliance is the extent to which patients follow the health advice they receive. Health advice encompasses taking medication, lifestyle changes including a special diet or exercise program, attending follow-up appointments, etc. The interpretation of this term encompasses a mutually acceptable regimen based on the doctor's recommendation and the patient's willingness and ability to follow the recommendation. Compliance can fluctuate, most often declining over time to the point of discontinuation. The concept of compliance can be summarized as having three stages:

$$\text{Compliance} = \text{Acceptance} \rightarrow \text{Execution} \rightarrow \text{Persistence}$$

EXPLANATION

Compliance on the part of the patient is dependent on a series of factors that represent the burden of treatment. This burden encompasses adverse effects, the complexity of the treatment regimen (i.e., multiple dose times, requirements to avoid or take with food, diet change, etc), as well as capacity to perform the tasks. The patient's readiness and willingness to undertake the treatment or lifestyle change separates patients into four broad categories (Cramer & Spilker 1991):

- Noncompliers: Those who do not accept the diagnosis and need for treatment at this time.
- Partial compliers: Those who accept the diagnosis and need for treatment but cannot fulfill the recommended actions sufficiently to reach targeted improvements in their health.
- Over-compliers: Those who take more than the recommended amount of medication or who diet or exercise in excess. (These patients are rare.)
- Adequate compliers: Those who follow the health advice adequately (i.e., enough medication, diet, exercise to improve or control their medical disorder).

## VALUE AND USE

Partial compliance and noncompliance are important considerations for several reasons.

1. The target outcome can be affected as much by compliance as by the selection of treatment.
   - Noncompliance means that the patient's health will not improve and will probably worsen. This can result in costly short- or long-term medical care.
   - Partial compliance means that the patient's health is not adequately managed. This can result in a stepped-care spiral into ever more complex and costly treatments that might not have been necessary if the patient had followed the initial regimen.
   - In contrast, adequate compliers do not necessarily need to take 100% of doses, diet, or exercise to achieve the desired results. Health care providers need to understand both the limitations of their knowledge to determine the optimum dose or therapy for an individual and the patient's ability to follow the regimen completely. Electronic monitoring of dosing has demonstrated that there is no magic number that represents the appropriate compliance rate for all patients or all disorders. The frequently quoted threshold of 80% compliance has no meaning unless it has been determined for the specific medication and target outcome.

2. Inadequate compliance may result in high follow-up costs during stepped care. Increased costs are incurred with extra outpatient visits, diagnostic tests to determine the reason for treatment failure, hospital admissions if the condition worsens, decreased work productivity, increased family burden, or increased mortality.

3. Inadequate compliance may result in a waste of resources if prescriptions for medications have been filled but not used. When the doctor who is

unaware of the degree of compliance with the regimen thinks that the medication has not been effective, higher doses, alternative drugs, or multiple drugs are prescribed.

4. The sequelae of inadequate compliance affect database assessments of resource utilization. Poor treatment outcomes result in increased costs that cannot be separated into costs for adequate compliers versus partial or noncompliers.

ISSUES

1. Methods to measure compliance
   - The standard methods of asking the patient, counting unused tablets, or observing the prescription refill rate all have inherent flaws. The gold standard of compliance measurement is electronic monitoring.
   - Various devices (e.g., bottle cap, inhaler, and liquid dispenser monitors) are available that collect continuous data based on dosing (Cramer 1995). The data can be downloaded to a computer for display. The data describe the dates and times of doses taken, a pattern of doses taken and missed, and calculations of overall compliance rates. The devices are widely used in clinical trials and in some clinical care situations.

2. Methods to improve compliance
   - Various measures can be taken to improve compliance. Simple methods include changing the form of administration (e.g., from multiple doses to once-daily administration), improving patient information (e.g., in the form of an educational material, consultation with a nurse, dietitian, etc.), and using a compliance enhancement program.
   - The most direct method of improving compliance is to assess actual compliance using electronic monitoring. This is cost-effective when the patient is not responding to standard treatment. Avoidance of costly stepped care makes electronic monitoring economical. Electronic data can be used in a "feedback system" designed to allow patients and clinicians to share information such that the patient is unlikely to feel judged or disparaged (Cramer & Rosenheck 1999). Patients can observe their patterns of dose-taking and omissions. Patients and clinicians can discuss events that were exacerbated because of missed doses. The feedback often is useful in designing therapy. The most common feature is the avoidance of dose or drug change based on the erroneous assumption that the drug failed. The electronic data demonstrate that insufficient doses were taken to provide an effective outcome.

3. Effects of compliance in economic evaluations
   - Currently, inadequate compliance is only a peripheral issue in economic evaluations. Part of the reason is because obtaining information from a database is difficult and time-consuming, and not enough reliable data are available. Another reason is that efficacy data from clinical trials deliberately exclude considerations of the natural environment. There-

fore, data from idealized trial conditions are not sufficient to evaluate the economic profitability of a medical service, as its actual effectiveness in practice is usually reduced by poor compliance. If, for example, a drug has proven efficacy, but in actual clinical practice some patients do not take it as prescribed because it has an unpleasant taste or is time-consuming to take, then the drug's actual effectiveness and, therefore, its potential economic advantage over other drugs are reduced. A third reason for lack of data is the limited use of electronic monitoring in clinical trials or general practice. If continuous electronic compliance monitoring was widely used within a health care system, the difference between a treatment failure and a patient's failure to take the treatment could be differentiated (Sullivan et al 1990).

- Measuring compliance is difficult, as it is dependent on the cooperation of the patient. Indirect methods such as reports written by the patients themselves or measurements of drug wastage are not precise enough for the purposes of most studies. On the other hand, direct methods (e.g., using marker substances or blood serum analyses) are very expensive and often unpleasant for the patient. The use of modern microchip technology to record when drugs are administered (e.g., built into metered aerosol inhalers) could help in the future to obtain more accurate data about time and frequency of drug administration.

The methodology of electronic monitoring has become the gold standard for compliance assessment in clinical research. Additional work is needed to define the implications of partial compliance in outcomes (Urquhart 1999).

BIBLIOGRAPHY

Cramer JA. Microelectronic systems for monitoring and enhancing patient compliance with medication regimens. *Drugs*. 1995;49:321–327.

Cramer JA, Rosenheck R. Enhancing medication compliance for people with serious mental disease. *J Nerv Mental Dis*. 1999;187:53–54.

Cramer JA, Spilker B, eds. *Patient Compliance in Medical Practice and Clinical Trials*. New York: Raven Press; 1991.

Sullivan SD, Kreling DH, Hazlet TH. Non-compliance with medication regimens and subsequent hospitalization: A literature analysis and cost of hospitalization analysis. *J Res Pharm Econ*. 1990;2:19–33.

Urquhart J. Pharmacoeconomic consequences of variable patient compliance with prescribed drug regimens. *Pharmacoeconomics*. 1999;15:217–228.

# Conjoint Analysis

## BRIEF DEFINITION

**Conjoint analysis** is a method for establishing the relative importance of different attributes in the provision of a good or a service.

## EXPLANATION

Conjoint analysis is a technique specifically designed to establish what factors influence the demand for different commodities and, thereby, which combinations of such attributes in products are preferred by consumers. Conjoint analysis is used to estimate the relative importance of the individual attributes; the willingness to trade between different attributes; and the total satisfaction or utility scores for different combinations of attributes.

There are five stages in the design of a conjoint analysis study:

1. Establishing the attributes, or the key features or characteristics, of the service or good. For example, in the treatment of laryngeal cancer, attributes could include speech quality and years of life.

2. Assigning levels to the attributes. The levels must be plausible, actionable and capable of being traded off. For example, two, four, or six years of life might be added by a particular treatment.

3. Determining the scenarios to present. Individuals are presented with hypothetical scenarios that combine different levels of attributes.

4. Establishing preferences. Preferences for scenarios are obtained by surveying patients/service users/members of the community.

5. Analysis of data. This involves identifying the relationship between the attributes and preferences using statistical regression analysis.

## VALUE AND USE

Conjoint analysis is a useful method for incorporating consumer preferences into decision making in health care systems. It can be used as an alternative to the standard gamble, time trade-off, and willingness-to-pay methods to evaluate health state preferences. Conjoint analysis can also be used in cost-benefit analysis to obtain willingness-to-pay values indirectly. By including different amounts of money as an attribute (known as the "cost attribute"), estimates of willingness to pay for changes in levels of the attributes of importance can be derived.

Conjoint analysis has been widely used in market research, transport economics, and environmental economics, but so far has had limited application in health economics. An example of the application of conjoint analysis in health care research has been to elicit information with regard to whether patients would prefer to receive treatment in local clinics with longer waiting times or to attend a centrally provided service with shorter waiting times.

## ISSUES

The conjoint analysis has been widely used in market research, transport economics and environmental economics, but so far has had limited application in health economics. However, studies show that conjoint analysis is an approach that circumvents well-known scaling problems of the standard gamble approach and the time trade-off technique. More research about the validity of the data needs to be done.

BIBLIOGRAPHY

Maas A, Stalpers L. Assessing utilities by means of conjoint measurement: an application in medical decision analysis. *Med Decis Making.* 1992;12:288–297.

McIntosh E, Donaldson C, Ryan M. Recent advances in the methods of cost-benefit analysis in health care—matching the art to the science. *Pharmacoeconomics.* 1999;15:357–367.

Szeinbach SL, Barnes JH, McGhan WF. Using conjoint analysis to evaluate health state preferences. *Drug Inf J.* 1999;33:849–858.

# Contingent Valuation
## Willingness to Pay

### BRIEF DEFINITION

**Contingent valuation** (CV) methodology is one way of simulating a missing market. The purpose is to determine an individual's maximum **willingness to pay** (WTP) (*see term:* Welfare Economics) for some good that usually does not have a market price (e.g., a health improvement) through hypothetical survey questions.

### EXPLANATION

Willingness to pay can be used as a measure of the strength of an individual's preferences. It has a clear foundation in economic theory and is here often referred to as compensating variation, or the maximum amount of money that can be taken from an individual after having provided a good while still leaving him or her at the same level of utility as before providing the good. Empirically, WTP can be measured either by revealed or by stated preferences. There exist several stated preference techniques, and contingent valuation is one of them. CV methodology is a way of simulating a missing market where an individual expresses his or her valuation for a good, contingent on a certain scenario. It thus seeks to determine individuals' maximum WTP for some (usually nonmarketed) good through hypothetical survey questions. The technique was originally developed to estimate the value of environmental changes, and most studies have so far been carried out in the environmental field. However, it has also been used for measuring the benefits of traffic safety, the value of life, and the value of health improvements.

### VALUE AND USE

Two approaches of determining WTP have been used in CV studies: elicitation of individuals' maximum WTP, and dichotomous choice (DC) questions. Techniques to determine an individual's maximum WTP include open-ended questions (in which the respondents are asked to directly state their maximum WTP), the so-called "bidding-game" (where respondents are given a first price for the good that is either accepted or rejected, and then the price is raised or lowered until the maximum WTP is reached), and the payment-card technique (where individuals choose a WTP amount from a range of suggested amounts on a card). Practically, open-ended questions can suffer from nonresponse (likely to occur due to responder difficulty with the structure of the question), the bidding game can introduce starting point bias (i.e., the maximum WTP depends on the first bid in the bidding game), and the payment-card method can cause range bias (respondents are influenced by the range of bids).

With DC questions, each respondent accepts or rejects only one price for the good, and each individual's maximum WTP will thus not be estimated. This structure more closely mimics consumer decisions, in which respondents accept or reject fixed prices. By varying the price (or the WTP bid) in different subsamples, it is possible to estimate an aggregate demand function for the good (where the idea is that a higher WTP bid is followed by a lower probability of answering "yes"). The mean WTP can then be calculated as the area under the aggregate demand curve, and the median WTP is the WTP in which probability of a "yes" answer is one-half, as shown in the figure. Starting point bias is avoided here, and response rates are usually higher. Drawbacks include the need for a usually larger sample size and that the entire aggregate demand function seldom is captured (i.e., there is rarely a bid that everyone accepts and a bid that everyone rejects), which makes the assumptions of the functional form very important. The DC approach has been recommended by an expert panel appointed by the National Oceanic and Atmospheric Administration to assess the validity of the CV method in the environmental field, and in recent years this approach also has gained some popularity within the field of health economics.

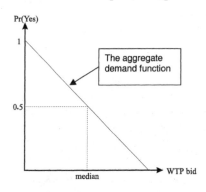

Overall, the strengths of the CV method are many: having a clear measure of the strength of an individual's preferences, expressed in monetary terms that can be used in a cost-benefit analysis, means that the decision rule becomes much simpler.

## ISSUES

Bias problems other than those stated above include scope effects (i.e., that the amount of the good or the size of the health effect should, but does not always seem to, matter, indicating that the response could be more a general approval than a real valuation) and hypothetical bias (i.e., that the stated WTP overestimates the real WTP). An individual's willingness to pay is constrained by his or her ability to pay; thus, if there are outcomes and programs of interest to the wealthy, they will receive higher WTP amounts than those of interest to the poor. Many see this as a serious flaw in the WTP approach. Political issues, such as whether health effects should be expressed in monetary terms at all and whether decision makers care about these kinds of benefits, also exist.

BIBLIOGRAPHY

Johannesson M. *Theory and Methods of Economic Evaluation of Health Care.* Dordrecht, The Netherlands: Kluwer Academic Publishers, 1996.

Kartman B, Stålhammar NO, Johannesson M. Valuation of health changes with the contingent valuation method: a test of scope and question order effects. *Health Econ.* 1996;5:531–541.

Liljas B, Blumenschein K. On hypothetical bias and calibration in cost-benefit studies. *Health Policy.* 2000;52:53–70.

# Cost-Benefit Analysis
## Cost-Benefit Ratio

BRIEF DEFINITION

**Cost-benefit analysis** (CBA) is an analytical technique derived from economic theory that enumerates and compares the net costs of a health care intervention with the benefits that arise as a consequence of applying that intervention. For this technique, both the net costs and the benefits of the health intervention are expressed in monetary units.

EXPLANATION

A health program is always compared against some alternative. The alternative may be an alternative intervention or it may be no treatment. The benefit of the intervention is the improved health outcomes as compared to the outcomes that would have been obtained with the alternative. The outcomes can include not only traditional patient outcomes but also option values (the benefit of having a treatment available just in case it is needed) and altruistic values (the benefit of seeing the health of others improve). The improved health outcomes are valued in monetary units, often by willingness to pay. The net cost of the intervention is the cost of the treatment and its follow-up (drugs, physicians, hospitals, home care, patient and family costs, costs of lost productivity, possibly costs of other kinds of lost time, etc.) less the cost of the treatment and follow-up with the alternative.

The bottom line of the analysis is the net benefit, which is the benefit minus the net cost (*see term:* Net Benefit). The net benefit is the basic decision criterion in CBA. If the net benefit is positive, the generally accepted decision rule is to fund the intervention.

Sometimes analyses compute the **cost-benefit ratio**, or alternatively, the benefit-cost ratio. This is just a ratio of the net cost figure and the benefit figure. However, the ratio is flawed as a decision criterion and its use is not recommended.

Cost benefit analysis takes a societal perspective and attempts to include all relevant costs and outcomes; however, the calculation of the indirect costs is sometimes controversial.

## VALUE AND USE

There are two major advantages of cost-benefit analysis, one of which is unique. First, like cost-utility analysis, it allows comparison of programs or interventions with entirely different outcomes. Thus it is possible to compare two completely unrelated programs strictly on a monetary basis. The economic decision rule is to choose the drug or treatment with the highest net benefit. Second, cost-benefit analysis is unique in being the only technique that has a definitive, self-contained decision rule for evaluating single interventions. If the net benefit of the intervention is positive, the intervention should be funded.

Cost-benefit analysis is not often used to compare drugs or alternative medical therapies because of ethical concerns related to placing a monetary value on human livelihood and to the methodologies used to assign such values.

## ISSUES

A key disadvantage of this type of analysis is the difficulty of converting or translating nonmonetary clinical and quality-of-life outcomes, such as lives or years saved, into monetary units. Moreover, the usual method of making this translation, willingness to pay, raises serious ethical issues because the method gives greater weight to the preferences of the wealthy. Thus this technique has not been widely used in health policymaking.

Most cost-benefit analyses are based on a model and require significant assumptions. Thus, it becomes important to validate the model assumptions and to determine the robustness of the results through sensitivity analysis.

## BIBLIOGRAPHY

Johannesson M, Weinstein MC. Designing and conducting cost-benefit analyses. In: Spilker B, ed. *Quality of Life and Pharmacoeconomics in Clinical Trials*. Philadelphia: Lippincott-Raven; 1996.

Robinson R. Cost-benefit analysis. *BMJ*. 1993;307:924–926.

Sloan FA. *Valuing Health Care: Costs, Benefits, and Effectiveness of Pharmaceuticals and other Medical Technologies*. Cambridge, UK: Cambridge University Press; 1995.

# Cost-Comparison Analysis
## Cost-Identification Analysis

## BRIEF DEFINITION

A **cost-comparison analysis** compares only the costs associated with two or more alternative health care treatments or interventions.

## EXPLANATION

A cost-comparison study is an analysis that enumerates all the costs, but not the consequences or other outcomes, of two or more health care treatments or interventions. The particular costs included in a study will be determined based on study perspective, available information, and relative magnitude of cost components. The process of identifying all the costs and their relative importance is often called a **cost-identification analysis**. It is important to ensure that all costs refer to the same base year. Costs from prior years need to be inflated to the base year using an appropriate price index. Future costs need to be discounted (*see term:* Discounting) back to the base year to establish their present value. The choice of costs measured needs to be consistently applied to all arms of a study.

VALUE AND USE

Cost-comparison studies often summarize their findings as a bottom-line figure. Decision makers often prefer this type of recommendation and/or conclusion and frequently focus on the budgetary impact of new treatments or interventions.

ISSUES

There are two main issues. With respect to the costing itself, areas of uncertainty include techniques for allocating shared overhead costs, discounting, and annuitization of capital expenditures. Fixed and variable costs as well as one-time and repetitive costs need to be dealt with carefully to ensure accuracy of the final result.

The other issue is that many people feel that it is inappropriate to consider the costs without regard to the benefits of treatments or interventions. One possible exception is if the two treatments or interventions are considered "equivalent." However, there is active debate over the appropriate use of cost-minimization studies and the ability of analysts to determine whether two treatments are "equivalent." The greatest issue is in devising guidelines on the exact meaning and proof of equivalency.

BIBLIOGRAPHY

Drummond MF, O'Brien B, Stoddart GL, et al. *Methods for the Economic Evaluation of Health Care Programmes.* 2nd ed. New York: Oxford University Press; 1997.
UK/US Purchasers Group. *Better Information, Better Outcomes.* New York: Milbank Memorial Fund, 2000.

# Cost-Consequence Analysis

BRIEF DEFINITION

A **cost-consequence analysis** compares the health intervention of interest to one or more relevant alternatives, listing the cost components and various outcomes of each intervention separately. This type of economic analysis does not indicate the relative importance of the components listed and leaves it to the decision maker to form his or her own view.

## EXPLANATION

A cost-consequence study is an economic analysis that makes few assumptions and places the greatest burden on the user of the analysis. The analysis does not combine the costs and consequences of the interventions. Each user must be able to integrate a disparate list of costs and outcomes of the various alternatives and reach an independent conclusion. Cost-consequence studies are based on the premise that the users of the study have the knowledge and experience to make value judgments for the trade-offs.

A cost-consequence study provides a comprehensive presentation of the cost and value of the intervention. It is a listing of all the relevant costs and outcomes or consequences of the interventions and may include the following components (*see term:* Cost – Health Economics):

- Direct medical costs
- Direct nonmedical costs
- Indirect costs (time costs, productivity costs)
- Health-related quality-of-life impact
- Utility impact
- Clinical outcomes (including side effects, adverse events)

The table below is an example of a cost-consequence analysis. Preferably these outcomes should be for the complete duration of the health condition. The ideal cost-consequence analysis would include all possible health outcomes or consequences. Presenting all possible costs and consequences allows decision makers the ability to determine the intervention's likely impact on their budgets and on the health of their patients.

## VALUE AND USE

The presentation of an array of output measures is a useful approach in presenting information to decision makers. Cost-consequence studies contain a wide range of health care resource utilization, costs, and outcome data. The availability of this breadth of data offers two advantages. First, it allows users to select whatever resources, costs, or outcomes are essential to make their decision. Secondly, the users may choose to use this data as a basis for other commonly employed types of economic analysis, such as cost-effectiveness analysis.

## ISSUES

The primary issue concerning cost-consequence studies is that they do not prescribe a weighting system of the relative importance of different costs and consequences. Since this information is provided in a disaggregated format, decision makers must devise their own weighting system to determine whether any health benefits associated with the new intervention are worth any extra costs incurred. Decisions made at the individual decision-maker level might not always be in the patients' or society's best interest.

Example of a Cost Consequence Table

|  | Intervention A | | Intervention B | |
| --- | --- | --- | --- | --- |
|  | Units | Costs | Units | Costs |
| **Direct medical costs** | | | | |
| Intervention A/B | | | | |
| Other medications/interventions | | | | |
| Physician Office Visits | | | | |
| ER visits | | | | |
| Hospitalizations | | | | |
| Home Care | | | | |
| **Direct non-medical costs** | | | | |
| Transportation | | | | |
| Paid caregiver time | | | | |
| **Indirect non-medical costs** | | | | |
| Patient time missed from work | | | | |
| Unpaid caregiver time off from work | | | | |
| **Symptom impact** | | | | |
| Patient distress days | | | | |
| Patient disability days | | | | |
| **Adverse Events** | | | | |
| Serious adverse events | | | | |
| Moderate adverse events | | | | |
| Mild adverse events | | | | |
| **Health-related Quality of Life impact** | | | | |
| Quality adjusted life years | | | | |
| Quality of life profile | | | | |

Reprinted with permission. © Adis International. Mauskopf JA, Paul JE, Grant DM, et al. The role of cost-consequence analysis in healthcare decision-making. *Pharmacoeconomics* 1998;13(3):277–288.

BIBLIOGRAPHY

Drummond MF, O'Brien B, Stoddart GL, et al. *Methods for the Economic Evaluation of Health Care Programmes.* 2nd ed. New York: Oxford University Press; 1997.

Gold MR, Siegel JE, Russell LB, et al. *Cost-Effectiveness in Health and Medicine.* New York: Oxford University Press; 1996.

Mauskopf JA, Paul JE, Grant DM, et al. The role of cost-consequence analysis in health care decision-making. *Pharmacoeconomics.* 1998;13:277–288.

# Cost-Effectiveness Acceptability Curve

## BRIEF DEFINITION

The **cost-effectiveness acceptability curve** (CEAC) plots the probability that one treatment is more cost-effective than another, as a function of the threshold willingness to pay for one additional unit of efficacy. The CEAC is a graphical expression of the cost-effectiveness comparison between two treatments (*see term:* Cost-Effectiveness Analysis).

EXPLANATION

Let the difference in mean costs between Treatment 2 and Treatment 1 be denoted by $\Delta_C$, and let the difference in mean efficacy (or effectiveness) between Treatment 2 and Treatment 1 be $\Delta_E$. Then the familiar incremental cost-effectiveness ratio (ICER) for Treatment 2 against Treatment 1 is $\Delta_C/\Delta_E$. The ICER is traditionally compared with a threshold willingness to pay for a unit of efficacy (such as quality adjusted life-years saved) $K$, such that if the ICER is less than $K$ then Treatment 2 should be accepted as more cost-effective than Treatment 1. However, there are difficulties with this approach to evaluating cost-effectiveness, and an alternative approach based on net benefits is increasingly preferred in practice.

The net monetary benefit of Treatment 2 against Treatment 1 is defined to be $K \Delta_E - \Delta_C$, while the net health benefit is $\Delta_E - \Delta_C/K$. They differ only in that the net monetary benefit is expressed in units of money while the net health benefit is expressed in units of efficacy. Both have the property that they are positive if, and only if, Treatment 2 is more cost-effective than Treatment 1.

In practice, we do not know the true values of either $\Delta_E$ or $\Delta_C$, and have only estimates of these quantities. The key measure then of whether Treatment 2 is more cost-effective than Treatment 1 is the probability that the net benefit is positive, that is: $Q(K) = \Pr(K \Delta_E - \Delta_C > 0) = \Pr(K \Delta_E > \Delta_C)$. Another complication is the fact that it is rare in health economics for the threshold willingness to pay $K$ to be known unambiguously. Consequently, it is useful to look at this probability $Q(K)$ for a range of values of $K$. The cost-effectiveness acceptability curve (CEAC), originally defined by Van Hout et al. (1994), encapsulates this thinking by plotting $Q(K)$ against $K$. An example is shown in Figure 1.

The CEAC gives a graphical description of the cost-effectiveness comparison between Treatment 2 and Treatment 1. If, over the range of plausible values of $K$, it is always well above a probability 0.5, then it is probable that Treatment 2 is more cost-effective than Treatment 1. In Figure 1, $Q(K)$ is above 0.7 (70%) for all $K$, and so the balance of evidence is quite firmly in favor of Treatment 2 being more cost-effective than Treatment 1.

If a higher degree of proof is desired, we see that $Q(K)$ exceeds 90% for all $K$ greater than 2000. Thus, if a health care provider is definitely willing to pay at least 2000 (in appropriate currency) for one unit of efficacy, then there is strong evidence that Treatment 2 is more cost-effective than Treatment 1.

Notice that Figure 1 plots $K$ on a logarithmic scale—this generally makes it easier to show the CEAC over its full range. Notice also that $Q(K)$ is not necessarily either an increasing or a decreasing function of $K$.

The simplest way to think about the CEAC is in terms of rotating the sloping line in the cost-effectiveness plane, shown in Figure 2. The line has slope $K$, and the probability of positive net benefit is always the probability that the true cost-effectiveness point $(\Delta_E, \Delta_C)$ lies *below* the line. When $K = 0$, the line is horizontal, and the CEAC is therefore the probability that Treatment 2 is cheaper than Treatment 1. As $K$ increases toward infinity, the line rotates to become vertical and the

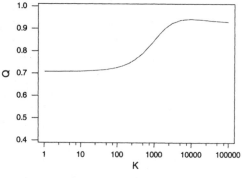

Figure 1.  A sample CEAC

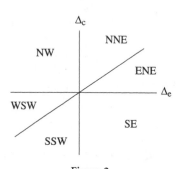

Figure 2.
The cost-effectiveness plane

CEAC is then the probability that Treatment 2 is more effective. At all intermediate values of $K$, the CEAC represents a balance between cost and efficacy.

### VALUE AND USE

The CEAC is in many ways the most helpful expression of the relative cost-effectiveness comparison between two treatments.

It should be noted that although usually defined as described above in terms of cost-effectiveness, the CEAC is equally valid and valuable in contexts generally called cost-utility or cost-benefit analyses in health economics. We have referred to $\Delta_E$ as the mean difference in efficacy, but it could equally well be in units of utility, for example QALYs, or some other measure of benefit.

Since it is defined in terms of probabilities, the CEAC will be computed through an appropriate statistical analysis. This might be in the context of a clinical trial of cost-effectiveness (in which both costs and efficacy/utility are measured or derived at the individual patient level). It might also arise in the context of economic modeling. In economic models, we invariably have some input parameters whose values are not known precisely, and it is then important to assess the sensitivity of model outputs to variations in those parameters. Probabilistic sensitivity analysis proceeds by assigning probability distributions to represent the uncertainty in these inputs, and thereby derives probability distributions for outputs such as $\Delta_E$ or $\Delta_C$. It is then natural to express the uncertainty about cost-effectiveness through a CEAC.

### ISSUES

Formally, the CEAC only has meaning within a Bayesian analysis (*see term:* Bayesian Analysis). This is because it is based on $Q(K)$, which involves attributing probabilities to unknown parameters. Parameters cannot be random variables and cannot have probability distributions within the frequentist approach to statistics. A frequentist analog of the CEAC has been defined by Löthgren and Zethraeus (2001), but the most natural formulation of the CEAC is its original Bayesian expression.

BIBLIOGRAPHY

Löthgren M, Zethraeus N. Definition, interpretation and calculation of cost-effectiveness acceptability curves. *Health Econ.* 2001;9:623–630.

O'Hagan A, Stevens JW, Montmartin J. Inference for the cost-effectiveness acceptability curve and cost-effectiveness ratio. *Pharmacoeconomics.* 2000;17:339–349.

Van Hout BA, ALM J, Gordon GS, Rutten F. Costs, effects and C/E ratios alongside a clinical trial. *Health Econ.* 1994;3:309–319.

# Cost-Effectiveness Analysis
Incremental Cost-Effectiveness Ratio
Reference Case

## BRIEF DEFINITION

**Cost-effectiveness analysis** is a systematic method of comparing two or more alternative programs by measuring the costs and consequences of each. A distinguishing feature of cost-effectiveness analysis is that the consequences (health outcomes) of all the programs to be compared must be measured in the same common units—natural units related to the clinical objective of the programs (e.g., symptom-free days gained, cases prevented, patients improved, life years gained). If there are just two alternative programs, their difference in cost (incremental cost) is compared to their difference in outcomes (incremental effect) by dividing the former by the latter. This ratio is known as the **incremental cost-effectiveness ratio** (ICER). If there are more than two alternatives, programs are compared on a systematic pair-wise basis using their ICERs.

## EXPLANATION

The major analytic techniques of health economic evaluation and of pharmacoeconomics are cost-minimization analysis, cost-effectiveness analysis, cost-utility analysis, cost-benefit analysis, and cost-consequence analysis (*see terms*: Cost-Benefit Analysis, Cost-Consequence Analysis, Cost-Minimization Analysis, Cost-Utility Analysis, Pharmacoeconomics,). All are similar in how they measure costs. The differences among the techniques are how the consequences or health outcomes are measured. In cost-minimization analysis, all health outcomes are assumed equal across all alternatives. In cost-effectiveness analysis a single, common unit of health outcome in natural units is used across all alternatives. In cost-utility analysis, utility scores are used to determine quality-adjusted life years gained, and this is used as the common outcome across all alternatives. In cost-benefit analysis, all outcomes are converted to their monetary equivalent, and money units become the common currency to compare across the alternatives. Some authors do not separate out cost-utility analysis as a different technique but include it as a special case of cost-effectiveness analysis. In this book of terms, cost-utility analysis is considered one of the five major analytic techniques (not a special case of cost-effective analysis). In cost-consequence analysis all costs and all outcomes are compared without indicating relative importance of each.

Cost-effectiveness analysis can be undertaken from different perspectives depending upon the needs of the decision makers. The most comprehensive perspective is the societal perspective in which all costs are included no matter to whom they occur. This would include all health care costs, all relevant non-health care costs (e.g., education, justice), all productivity costs (e.g., lost work time), and all patient and family costs (e.g., travel, baby sitting, home modifications, time of family caregivers, lost patient nonworking time). More restricted perspectives include the health care system, a particular payer (e.g., managed care, third-party insurer), a particular institution (e.g., hospital), or the patient.

A single outcome measure must be selected for all the programs to be compared at one time with cost-effectiveness analysis. Typically this is the primary clinical outcome measure for the programs being compared (e.g., cases detected, symptom-free days, percent serum cholesterol reduction, life years gained). Ideally, outcome measures should relate to a final outcome such as life-years gained rather than to an intermediate clinical measure such as percent serum cholesterol reduction. If intermediate outcomes must be used, it is important to establish the link between such outcomes and final outcomes, or to show that such intermediate outcomes themselves have value.

Costs and outcomes that occur in the future must be discounted to their equivalent present value using an established discount rate (*see term:* Discounting).

Cost-effectiveness analysis attempts to determine the true costs and outcomes that would occur in the real world, not in the artificial world of clinical trials. Thus, if effectiveness data is taken from clinical trials, some authors use the term "cost-efficacy analysis" to indicate that the outcomes represent efficacy rather than effectiveness. Efficacy refers to the outcomes achieved in the highly controlled environment of clinical trials. Effectiveness represents outcomes achieved in the real world.

Cost-effectiveness studies may be prospective studies or modeled studies. In prospective studies patients are randomized to the competing alternatives and costs, and outcomes are collected over the duration of the study. Ideally, these should be effectiveness (pragmatic) trials as opposed to efficacy trials. If the latter, appropriate adjustments should be made (e.g., compliance) to convert to the real world. In modeled studies, outcomes are often taken from clinical trials or from a meta-analysis or systematic review of trials, and costs are taken from real world experience.

After determining the costs and effects of each program, the programs are compared using the cost-effectiveness ranking algorithm (*see term:* Dominance). It consists of ranking the programs in order of their costs, eliminating those that are dominated by simple dominance, computing the ICERs, eliminating those that are dominated by extended dominance, computing the final ICERs, and interpreting the results.

Finally, the uncertainties in the data and in the methodologic assumptions should be investigated by sensitivity analysis to determine the impact on the results.

## VALUE AND USE

Cost-effectiveness analysis is the most widely used of the techniques of health economic evaluation and pharmacoeconomics. It is unequivocally central to the field. The literature is full of countless examples.

To enhance the comparability across different cost-effectiveness studies, the Panel on Cost-Effectiveness in Health and Medicine convened by the US Public Health Service recommended that all studies include a reference case. The reference case prescribes standard approaches (e.g., how to measure costs, how to measure effectiveness, use of quality-adjusted life years, whose preferences to use for quality-adjusting life years, use of 3% discount rate, how to deal with uncertainty, etc). The intent was that all studies should do a **reference case** analysis in addition to any other analyses desired by the study authors, and these reference cases, all done with comparable methods, would allow comparisons across different cost-effectiveness studies.

## ISSUES

Many cost-effectiveness analyses are performed from a restricted perspective: for example, the perspective of a particular payer. This may not lead to the best overall solution for the health care system, as it may lead merely to cost-shifting. For example, it can be cost-effective for a particular payer to off-load costs and problems onto some other part of the system. For this reason, the Panel on Cost-Effectiveness in Health and Medicine recommended that the reference case use a comprehensive societal perspective.

There are many issues related to costing, and these are taken up elsewhere in the costing sections of this book. One of the more contentious issues is how to cost lost time, both lost work time and lost nonwork time.

Although most methods guidelines, including the reference case guidelines of the US Panel, recommend discounting costs and effects at the same rate, this continues to be a contentious issue in some quarters, and one jurisdiction (the United Kingdom) mandates a lower discount rate for effects than costs.

## BIBLIOGRAPHY

Gold MR, Siegel JE, Russell LB, Weinstein MC. *Cost-Effectiveness in Health and Medicine.* New York: Oxford University Press; 1996.

Hunink M, Glasziou P, Siegel J, et al. *Decision-Making in Health and Medicine: Integrating Evidence and Values.* Cambridge, UK: Cambridge University Press; 2001.

Weinstein M, Stason W. Foundations of cost-effectiveness analysis for health and medical practices. *N Engl J Med.* 1977;296:716–721.

# Cost Measurement Methods

Human Capital Method
Friction Cost Method

Two methods of cost measurement are generally used by health care analysts: the **human capital method** and the **friction cost method**.

## Human Capital Method

BRIEF DEFINITION
The human capital method is a method of estimating productivity cost in the absence of market prices. This method estimates the value of human capital as the present value of an individual's future earnings.

EXPLANATION
As indicated by its name, the human capital method is used to obtain an estimate of the human capital of an individual. Human capital consists of individual assets such as knowledge, skills, and other characteristics contributing to the individual's ability to produce. Only assets that have been obtained by investment (e.g., education, work training, and health) contribute to human capital. Individual assets not acquired through investment, such as genetic characteristics, are not included in human capital.

VALUE AND USE
The lost productivity associated with death, illness, or injury using the human capital approach is the market value of that individual's future contribution to production if he or she had continued to be in full health. Hence, the method is used to estimate the indirect cost of illness. If a health care program can avoid the premature death, illness, or injury (i.e., by an investment in health) and if the investment cost is less than the loss in human capital, the program is worth undertaking according to the human capital method.

ISSUES
The underlying assumption that the human capital of an individual equals the individual's expected future productivity is rather unrealistic in many situations. One issue is the use of future earnings as a proxy for future production. In many cases future earnings do not reflect future production—housewives are good examples of this. Moreover, the human capital method is not consistent with general welfare economics since it does not take into account the value of leisure time and other activities. In addition, the human capital method has been criticized because of the underlying assumption that a worker cannot be replaced even if the unemployment rate is significantly high. The human capital method would in this respect overestimate the value of foregone production.

BIBLIOGRAPHY

Johansson PO. *Evaluating Health Risks—An Economic Approach.* Cambridge, UK: Cambridge
    University Press; 1995.
Mincer J. Investment in human capital and personal income distribution. *J Polit Econ.* 1958;
    66:281–302.
Pauly VM. Valuing health care benefits in money terms. In Sloan FA, ed. *Valuing Health Care.*
    Cambridge, UK: Cambridge University Press; 1996.

## Friction Cost Method

BRIEF DEFINITION

The friction cost method is a method of estimating productivity cost in the
absence of market prices. This method estimates the value of human capital as
another worker from the unemployment pool replaces the present value of a
worker's future earnings until the ill and absent worker returns or is replaced.

EXPLANATION

The friction cost method has been developed as an alternative approach to the
human capital method. Whereas the human capital method assigns the whole
value of an individual's future earnings as the indirect cost, the friction cost
method assigns only the value of the individual's future earnings until another
worker from the unemployment pool replaces the ill worker. As a consequence,
the friction cost is restricted to the short-term consequences of illness, injury,
or premature death. The short-term period is called the friction period and is
defined as the period needed to replace the sick worker. The length of this
period depends on the general unemployment level and on the efficiency of the
matching process between job seekers and vacancies. It also depends on factors
such as age, sex, and education.

VALUE AND USE

The loss in human capital due to illness, injury, or premature death is measured
as the estimated value of the lost production. The value of this lost production
is then used as an estimate of the indirect cost of illness.

ISSUES

Regardless of whether the human capital approach or the friction cost method
is used, the loss in human capital will be more or less the same in the short-
term perspective. However, in the long-term perspective the friction cost
method will result in a cost estimate lower than the human capital method. The
main reason for this is that the friction cost method, in contrast to the human
capital method, assumes that after the friction period the ill worker will be
replaced by a previously unemployed one, and therefore limits the cost of lost
production to the friction period. Hence, the friction cost method assumes that
illness, injuries, or premature deaths will not affect the total productivity follow-

ing the friction period. The controversial conclusion from this is the friction cost method suggests that illness, injuries, and premature deaths would reduce the total unemployment rate in the economy.

BIBLIOGRAPHY

Goeree R, O'Brien BJ, Blackhouse G, Agro K, Goering P. The valuation of productivity costs due to premature mortality: a comparison of the human-capital and friction-cost methods for schizophrenia. *The Can J Psychiatry.* 1999;44:455–463.

Johannesson M, Karlsson G. The friction cost method: a comment. *J Health Econ.* 1997;16,249–16,255.

Koopmanschap MA, Rutten FFH, van Ineveld BM, van Roijen L. The friction cost method for measuring indirect costs of disease. *J Health Econ.* 1995;14:171–189.

# Cost-Minimization Analysis

## BRIEF DEFINITION

**Cost-minimization analysis** (CMA) is a type of pharmacoeconomic analysis comparing two alternative therapies only in terms of costs because their outcomes (effectiveness and safety) are found to be or expected to be identical.

## EXPLANATION

The economic analysis of medical technologies, in general, and pharmaceutical therapies, in particular, is based on the principle of comparing alternatives in terms of costs and of health outcomes. The principal types of analyses—cost-consequence analysis, cost-minimization analysis, cost-effectiveness analysis, cost-utility analysis, and cost-benefit analysis (*see terms:* Cost-Benefit Analysis, Cost-Consequence Analysis, Cost-Effectiveness Analysis, Cost-Utility Analysis)—differ primarily in terms of how the health outcomes (i.e., items that are not included in costs) are assessed and measured. Because of the difficulties of measuring outcomes or effectiveness, the approaches differ primarily in how they handle this valuation. Cost-consequence analysis simply lists the consequences (survival impact, pain, quality of life, etc) for decision makers to consider and apply their own preferences and valuations. Cost-effectiveness analysis focuses on a single important outcome parameter, e.g., symptom-free months, and compares the alternatives as a ratio in terms of the incremental cost of any incremental gain in that effectiveness measure. Cost-utility analysis uses preference measurement techniques to convert the vector of consequences into a nonmonetary metric, such as quality-adjusted life year (QALY) or healthy-years equivalent (HYE) (*see terms:* Healthy-Years Equivalent [HYE], Quality-Adjusted Life Year [QALY]). The measure then becomes a ratio of the incremental cost per QALY gained (for example), which can be compared with other technologies for which this metric has been applied to the denominator. Cost-benefit analysis takes the further step of valuing the alternative health outcomes in monetary terms by applying valuation techniques such as willingness to pay or contingent valuation (*see term:* Contingent Valuation). The existence of these alternative methods to evaluating health outcomes is testimony to the difficulty of the task. Cost-minimization analysis has the conceptual advantage of avoiding this problem because the health outcomes are deemed or demonstrated to be equivalent; hence, the preferred alternative will be the least costly one.

## VALUE AND USE

In practical terms, the value and use of cost-minimization analysis is very limited for assessing new medical interventions, especially new pharmaceuticals. With the exception of generic drugs, most new compounds are expected to have at least a slightly different side effects profile, if not efficacy differential, simply by being a different molecular entity. In the case of generic copies, the health outcomes should be the same, so the comparison becomes a trivial comparison of drug acquisition costs.

Sometimes the term "CMA" is used in a loose, nontechnical sense to compare "me-too" drugs, slightly differing molecules with the same mechanism of action that produce clinical outcomes that are only slightly different, but identical for practical or measurable clinical purposes. One could say that comparing them is really a matter of cost minimization, viz, choosing the one with lower acquisition cost.

A more interesting analysis would be having two different drugs in the same class and with identical clinical endpoints for efficacy and safety, but with a different formulation, for example tablet versus intravenous infusion. The difference in costs of the two would involve more than just acquisition cost. The latter might require visits to providers that would require additional time and administration costs that need to be considered.

## ISSUES

From a practical decision-making point of view, it is certainly possible to think of drug comparisons, such as between me-too drugs, in which the clinical outcomes (i.e., efficacy and safety) would not be judged to be significantly different. In those situations, the comparison should logically focus on differences in costs of drug acquisition and administration and differences in nonmedical costs, such as the value of a patient's time. As Briggs and O'Brien (2001) elucidate, the limitations of CMA are underscored by considering its use in the economic evaluation of pharmaceuticals alongside clinical trials, which may not be powered to measure either clinical differences or cost differences. A trial could support the hypothesis of clinical (outcome) equivalence either when it was powered to demonstrate that or when it was underpowered to find a difference. In the former instance it would be proper to go ahead and apply statistical tests only to the measured cost difference. In the latter instance, such tests would be improper and could lead to the wrong decision. In these situations, the estimation of cost-effectiveness ratios with appropriate confidence intervals is a more reliable technique.

BIBLIOGRAPHY

Briggs AH, O'Brien BJ. The death of cost-minimization analysis? *Health Econ.* 2001;10:179–184.

Drummond MF, O'Brien B, Stoddart GL, et al. *Methods for the Economic Evaluation of Health Care Programmes.* 2nd ed. Oxford, UK: Oxford University Press; 1997.

Torrance GW, Seigel JE, Luce BR. Framing and designing the cost-effectiveness analysis. In: Gold MR, Siegel JE, Russell LB, et al. eds. *Cost-Effectiveness in Health and Medicine.* New York: Oxford University Press; 1996.

# Cost-of-Illness Study

## BRIEF DEFINITION

A **cost-of-illness study** (COI) or a cost-of-disease study aims to determine the total economic impact (cost) of a disease or health condition on society through the identification, measurement, and valuation of all direct and indirect costs. This form of study focuses on costs and does not address questions relating to treatment efficiency.

## EXPLANATION

COI studies provide an estimate (in monetary terms) of the total economic impact to society of a particular disease. Adopting such a societal viewpoint can include a measure of the financial burden falling onto different sectors of society including: the state or government (e.g., health and social welfare ministries), specific organizations or institutions (e.g., employers, health insurances, sickness funds), and individuals themselves with the condition.

Performing a COI study means adopting one of two main approaches to costing. The prevalence approach (the most commonly used) provides an estimate of the total annual cost associated with a disease. The approach provides an estimate of the lifetime costs of incident cases diagnosed in a given year. Within these overarching frameworks, individual component costs (i.e., direct, indirect) are addressed in different ways. Direct costs are calculated using either the "top-down" or "bottom-up" costing techniques or both. Indirect costs, associated with lost economic activity (i.e., the value of the output that is lost to an economy because people are too ill to work or die prematurely) are calculated using the human capital method (most common method) or the friction cost method (*see term:* Cost Measurement Methods). The choice of any specific methodology used is often determined by the data available to the investigator.

## VALUE AND USE

COI studies communicate to the reader a measure of the total expenditure (as well as the relative weighting of direct and indirect costs) spent on a particular disease (e.g., the use of health and social care services) in comparison to the scope of the health problem (i.e., epidemiological estimates of mortality and morbidity of the disease). Comparisons can theoretically be made across diseases (e.g., across chronic diseases such as asthma, diabetes, or arthritis or prevention programs such as breast cancer prevention) within a particular county or region or between countries. For example, Barnes et al reviewed the literature on cost-of-illness studies in asthma and compared direct and indirect costs across Europe, North America, and Australia.

COI studies have been controversial with respect to their use in resource prioritizing decisions. In addition, COI studies provide a market measure for the pharmaceutical industry with respect to assessing market volume potential (low to high) and treatment patterns of specific health problems and diseases.

## ISSUES

COI studies certainly raise the cost-consciousness of policymakers and provide a simple, single index of the burden of illness (total, direct, and indirect costs versus the scope of the health problem). However, both the choice of costing methodologies available to researchers (e.g., human capital vs friction cost to estimate indirect costs) and the use of the results of COI studies to aid resource prioritizing decisions remain contentious issues. Indirect costs often represent a large proportion of reported total costs in COI studies (an issue in itself), and can vary considerably depending on which approach is employed.

The argument that COI studies point to areas in which cost savings might be made (if a disease is eradicated or the burden lessened) is often unrealistic or at best overestimated. Decisions on the allocation of (scarce) resources should depend on the availability of treatment options, their cost, and their effectiveness. Although COI studies can provide a baseline against which new interventions can be assessed, this form of study provides very limited understanding of what health gains are attainable from specific treatment interventions and prevention programs for a given level of expenditure: that is, whether specific interventions are financially worthwhile. Cost-effectiveness, cost-utility, and cost-benefit analyses are required for this kind of analysis.

## BIBLIOGRAPHY

Barnes PJ, Jonsson B, Klim JB. The costs of asthma. *Eur Respir J.* 1996;9:636–642.
Drummond M. Cost of illness studies: A major headache? *Pharmacoeconomics.* 1992;2:1–4.
Rice DP. Cost of illness studies: fact or fiction. *Lancet.* 1994;344:1519–1520.

# Cost-Utility Analysis

## BRIEF DEFINITION

**Cost-utility analysis** (CUA) is a methodology of economic analysis that compares two or more alternative choices in terms of both their costs and their outcomes, where the outcomes are measured in units of utility or preference, often as a quality-adjusted life year (QALY) (*see term:* Quality-Adjusted Life Year [QALY]). The purpose of the analysis is to compare, using cost-effectiveness, two or more alternative choices in terms that are both clinically meaningful and can be compared with other economic analyses. Cost-utility analysis can be considered the "gold standard" methodology for evaluating the cost effectiveness of health care choices.

## EXPLANATION

Cost-utility analysis is a specific type of cost-effectiveness analysis (*see term:* Cost-Effectiveness Analysis) in which the denominator is measured in terms of quality-adjusted life years gained. This standard outcomes measurement is important because it allows cost-utility measures to be compared across studies and allows one to determine a level of "acceptable" cost utility for health care choices: that is, a "threshold level" of cost/QALY. In contrast, cost-effectiveness analyses that use an intermediate outcome as the denominator such as cost per infection cleared, or cost per cancer detected, cannot be compared with each other. Cost-benefit analysis that uses the human capital method to evaluate survival effects can be inequitable when comparing some groups, such as males and females, or the elderly and the young, as this measure depends on one's ability to earn income. CUA is a methodology that avoids these deficiencies of the other two methods. In addition, CUA has the advantage over other cost-effectiveness methodologies of including quality adjustments, which are especially important when two alternatives differ in their effects on the quality of life as well as on survival.

A cost-utility analysis is expressed in terms of a ratio of the incremental costs of two alternatives over the incremental quality-adjusted life years of the two alternatives. The result shows the cost of saving one quality-adjusted life year (cost/QALY) for that choice.

## VALUE AND USE

CUA is used to determine the relative value of alternative health care programs. It is similar to cost-effectiveness analysis except for its use of QALYs as the measurement of outcome in the denominator. Therefore the focus of this discussion is on the use of QALYs in a CUA, and one should refer to the entry on Cost-Effectiveness Analysis for more information.

The denominator in the cost/utility ratio is the incremental gain in QALYs comparing one program to another. The advantage of using QALYs as the outcome measure is that it allows comparability across all CUA studies. QALYs are a universal measure that can be applied to all patients and all diseases. In this way, QALYs provide the common metric that enables decision makers to compare CUA ratios across different studies. See the section on Quality-Adjusted Life Years for more details.

The quality weights for QALYs are based on individual preferences for different health states. These quality weights, or utilities, can be measured directly using time-consuming instruments such as standard gamble, time trade-off (*see terms:* Utility, Utility Measurement), or sometimes even with a visual analog scale.

The quality weights can also be provided more simply by using one of the multi-attribute utility indexes such as the Health Utilities Index, EuroQol EQ-5D, or Quality of Well-Being (*see term:* Health Utilities Index).

Alternatives to the use of the QALY for cost-utility analyses are also suggested. For example, the World Bank uses the disability-adjusted life year (DALY) (*see term:* Disability-Adjusted Life Year), and others suggest that a measure of healthy-year equivalents (*see term:* Healthy-Years Equivalent) is a more accurate reflection of utility than are QALYs. Most CUAs, however, are conducted using cost/QALY as the unit of measurement.

QALYs are calculated by summing the product of the survival years and the utility for each year of survival. If the survival year is spent in perfect health, that year is multiplied by one and therefore has a full value. However, if that year is spent in a health state specified with a 0.8 utility value, that year's survival is $1 \times 0.8$ or 0.8 QALY. If all 5 years of survival due to an intervention have a 0.8 utility value, the total QALY for that intervention (A) is calculated as $5 \times 0.8 = 4$ QALYs. If the alternative intervention B has the same survival of 5 years but with perfect health, then the calculation is $5 \times 1 = 5$ QALYs.

The incremental CUA of alternative B versus A is calculated as:

$$(\text{Cost B} - \text{Cost A})/(\text{QALY of B} - \text{QALY of A}).$$

If the cost of intervention B is $5000 and the cost of A is $4000, and if the QALYs of B are 5 and the QALYs of A are 4 (as described above) so that intervention B is more costly but also provides more QALYs, then the incremental CUA of B is $(\$5000 - \$4000)/(5 - 4) = \$1000/1$ QALY.

Therefore, it costs an additional $1000 per each additional QALY gained to choose alternative B over alternative A.

EXAMPLE

A cost-utility analysis to compare the use of interferon in stage II malignant melanoma patients who are positive for micrometastasis with a sentinel lymph node biopsy (SLN) are presented below in steps as an example.

1. Identify the two alternative decisions: Strategy A is not to test or treat anyone with interferon with stage II malignant melanoma, and Strategy B is to test everyone with SLN and treat all positives with high dose interferon.

2. Gather outcome data, utility data, and cost data: Clinical trial data is used

to assess survival at 5 years with the use or nonuse of interferon in stage II patients. A utility study which measured the utility of different health states with malignant melanoma and with and without interferon treatment is used to adjust survival to account for the effects of the side effects of interferon and the effects of the melanoma itself on subjects. Costs were estimated from a combination of the literature, Medicare costs, and locally derived costs.

3. Determine life expectancy, utility, and cost:

|  | Quality Adjusted Survival (years) | Costs |
|---|---|---|
| Strategy A: No test, no interferon | 3.06 | $18400 |
| Strategy B: SLN test, interferon to positives | 3.37 | $24200 |

4. Calculate the incremental CUA:

$$\text{CUA} = \frac{\text{Cost Strategy B} - \text{Cost Strategy A}}{\text{QALY Strategy B} - \text{QALY Strategy A}}$$

$$= \frac{\$24200 - \$18400}{3.37 - 3.06}$$

$$= \frac{5800}{0.31}$$

$$= \$18700 / \text{QALY}$$

5. Draw conclusions: Therefore it costs an additional $18700 per additional QALY saved if you choose to test all stage II patients with SLN and then treat those who are positive with high dose interferon treatment rather than not testing anyone and not providing any stage II patients with interferon treatment. This is below the often-used cut-off threshold of $50000 per QALY, and therefore strategy B is a cost-effective choice.

## ISSUES

Several issues are debated with respect to CUA and utilities. One is whether cost/QALY should be the "gold standard" for cost-effectiveness analyses. Although this type of analysis offers a standardization that allows comparisons across interventions, it may not measure equitably across all interventions. For example, it may be necessary to provide different cut-off threshold CUA values for chronic versus acute conditions.

Other issues important to CUA are those related to utility measurement itself. Different methods to measure the utility score produce different utility scores. Methods and instruments to measure utilities include both direct approaches, such as the standard gamble and time trade-off, and indirect approaches, such as the Health Utilities Index and EuroQol EQ-5D.

CUA includes both the length of life and the quality of life. In the early days of CUA, utility could only be incorporated in a study by undertaking time-consuming and difficult direct measurement. Accordingly, utility was often not included in the earliest cost-effectiveness studies or was not measured as accurately as is desirable. Thus in the early days there were more CEAs and fewer CUAs. More recently, simple multiattribute utility instruments have become available (e.g., Health Utilities Index, EuroQol EQ-5D, Quality of Well-Being) that can be readily added to virtually any study. Accordingly, CUAs are now becoming more common.

BIBLIOGRAPHY

Drummond MF, O'Brien BJ, Stoddart GL, Torrance GW. *Methods for the Economic Evaluation of Health Care Programmes*. 2nd ed. Oxford, UK: Oxford University Press; 1997.

Gold MR, Siegel JE, Russell LB, Weinstein MC. Cost-effectiveness in Health and Medicine. New York: Oxford University Press; 1996.

Wilson LS, Reyes CM, Lu C, et al. Modelling the cost-effectiveness of sentinel lymph node mapping and adjuvant interferon treatment for stage II melanoma. *Melanoma Res*. 2002;12:607–617.

# Cost – General

Fixed Cost
Variable Cost
Total Cost
Average Cost
Marginal Cost
Sunk Costs

BRIEF DEFINITION

Cost refers to the sacrifice of alternative benefits made when a given resource is used for any purpose (e.g., consumption or production).

EXPLANATION

As the saying goes, there is no free lunch. Any activity we undertake involves costs. The cost of engaging in an activity is the sum of all other benefits that can be generated by the same amount of resources taken away from us for this activity. It is commonly seen that the terms cost and opportunity cost (*see term:* Cost – Opportunity Cost) are used interchangeably. There are many subterms of costs. For example: **fixed cost, variable cost, total cost, average cost** and **marginal cost**. In health economics, cost is composed of direct cost and indirect cost when calculated from the societal perspective (*see term:* Cost – Health Economics).

Fixed cost is the type of cost that does not vary with the amount of output produced (typically, within one year) and generally includes investment such as equipment and land that cannot be obtained or traded in the short run. However, in the long run, fixed cost will vary when a firm has enough time to adjust its production strategy. Variable cost is composed of material expenses and wages that can change according to the amount of output produced. In the short run, total cost of production equals the sum of fixed cost and variable cost. Average cost is total cost divided by the quantity of output. Marginal cost refers to the extra cost of producing an additional unit of output.

## VALUE AND USE

Cost and benefit are the two most important factors considered by any decision makers for resource allocation. Costs can be measured in terms of any type of resource (e.g., time or food), but most commonly they are measured in terms of money. In calculating a cost, it is important not to double-count. For example, the time we spent watching a movie could have been used to play tennis or to write a paper, but not both. Therefore, it would not be correct to count both the forgone tennis game and the forgone paper as the cost of watching a movie.

When facing options that generate the same benefits with different costs, a rational person will choose the option with the lowest cost. Generally, if none of the options can generate more benefit than cost, this rational person will not take any option. To achieve an optimal point (where the profit is maximum or the loss is minimum), however, marginal cost and marginal revenue/benefit will be better indices. For a firm to maximize profit (or minimize loss), given no constraints, it should produce at the point where the marginal cost equals the marginal benefit—the optimal point. Note that when total cost equals total benefit it will only be break-even. For a consumer to obtain the maximum utility when the budget allows, he or she will continue to consume a good until the marginal utility equals the marginal cost.

## ISSUES

Note that "cost" is not "price." The market usually determines price. The process of determining the "price" of a good or service is usually more complicated than determining the "cost" because it varies in different types of market and depends on many factors (e.g., taxes, subsidies). For example, in a monopoly or oligopoly market (i.e., a market that only has one or very few sellers), the sellers can charge a price that is much higher than the product's cost.

When calculating the cost of an activity with a long duration or which occurred several years in the past, the cost should be converted (either discounted or inflated) to the present value with a properly chosen rate. When using cost data from different countries, a common currency should be chosen and exchange rates should be applied to convert the costs obtained in other countries to those based on that specific currency.

Sometimes a firm is better off producing outputs even if the average cost is higher than the market price. This possibility arises in a situation when the price is higher than the average variable cost, so the firm can cover some of the fixed costs and will not lose all of the investment made on capital goods. The investment in capital goods will become **sunk costs** when the firm stops production completely.

BIBLIOGRAPHY

Landsburg S. *Price Theory and Applications.* Cincinnati, Ohio: South-Western College Publishing; 1999.

Mansfield E. *Managerial Economics.* Philadelphia: W.W. Norton & Company, Inc; 1995.

# Cost – Health Economics

| | |
|---|---|
| Direct Cost | Ancillary Cost |
| Indirect Cost | Averted Cost |
| Intangible Cost | Incremental Cost |
| Acquisition Cost | Out-of-Pocket Cost |
| Allowable Cost | |

BRIEF DEFINITION

Cost in health economics refers to the resources consumed during the provision of health care.

EXPLANATION

There are generally three types of cost—direct, productivity (or indirect), and intangible. **Direct cost** refers to those resources whose consumption is wholly attributable to use of the health care intervention in question. Direct costs include resources such as physical goods, labor, and time. The term **indirect costs** is used differently in different disciplines; however, in pharmacoeconomics and outcomes research it generally refers to lost productivity (paid or unpaid) resulting from morbidity or mortality. Both direct and productivity costs are typically presented in monetary terms. **Intangible cost** refers to the pain and suffering imposed by disease and its treatment and are typically more difficult to quantify in monetary terms.

Resources used and their costs for the same intervention will vary when calculated from different perspectives (e.g., societal perspective or payer's perspective).

Several subterms related to costs in health economics:

**Acquisition cost:** the purchase price of a drug, device, or other health care intervention to an institution or a person. Acquisition cost for the same product or service typically varies depending on the purchaser and on the arrangements made between the manufacturer or provider of the service and the ultimate practitioner who delivers or provides the product to the patient.

**Allowable cost:** the charge for services rendered or supplies furnished by a health provider that qualify as expenses covered by the insurer or government payer.

**Ancillary cost:** the fee associated with additional services such as laboratory work, X-ray, and anesthesia that are performed prior to and/or secondary to a significant procedure.

**Averted cost:** a potential financial outlay (for resource utilization) that is avoided by using an alternative health care intervention, typically compared to standard care.

**Incremental cost:** the additional cost of a health care product or service compared to an alternative.

**Intangible cost:** costs assigned to the amount of suffering that occurs because of the disease or health care intervention. Increasingly these are being included in utility assessments.

**Out-of-pocket cost:** the portion of a payment paid for by an individual with his or her own money as opposed to the portion paid for by the insurer. For example, copayments and deductibles are out-of-pocket costs.

## VALUE AND USE

In any decision analysis model, cost is always one of the factors included while its counterfactor varies from benefit (in cost-benefit analysis), effectiveness (in cost-effectiveness analysis), and quality-adjusted life years or utility (in cost-utility analysis). While comparing two interventions that can achieve the same outcome, cost would be the only factor that a decision maker has to consider. Such analyses are often called cost-minimization analyses.

Two elements of estimating cost are: measurement of the quantities of resource used and the assignment of unit costs or prices. The measurement of quantities is generally relatively straightforward with the use of case report forms (in clinical trials), case notes, hospital records, or other data collection systems. Unit costs might not always be available and often vary across different regions, time periods, or providers.

Two common approaches to account indirect costs are through a human capital method or a friction cost method (*see term:* Cost Measurement Methods). The main difference between the two methods is that the friction cost method reduces the period of production loss to the period needed to replace the sick employee: the friction period.

## ISSUES

In addition to those issues covered above, several others have to be considered when calculating costs for health products or services:

1. How can costs be estimated for nonmarket items? Patient/family leisure time and volunteer time are major nonmarket resource inputs to health care programs. To estimate the costs of these types of resources, the market wage rate can be used as a proxy. One can argue, though, that the cost of leisure time lost could be anything from zero to average overtime earnings. For other nonmarket items, their costs can be estimated

through different economic techniques such as contingent valuation and conjoint analysis.

2.  How long should costs be tracked? This is up to the analyst so long as the result does not mislead the decision maker or user. The choice of follow-up period for estimating therapy-specific or disease-specific costs should not bias the analysis in favor of one intervention over another.

3.  What about inconsistency in estimating morbidity costs—in numerator or denominator? Under specific circumstances, it does not matter whether some costs (e.g., patient intangible costs, patient out-of-pocket productivity costs) are incorporated in the numerator (in dollar terms) or in the denominator (QALYs) of the cost/effectiveness ratio, as long as the practice is consistent.

BIBLIOGRAPHY

Drummond M, O'Brien B, Stoddart G, Torrance G. *Methods for the Economic Evaluation of Health Care Programmes.* New York: Oxford University Press; 1997.

Koopmanschap M, Rutten F. A practical guide for calculating indirect costs for disease. *Pharmacoeconomics.* 1999;10:460–466.

Gold M, Siegel J, Russell L, Weinstein M, eds. *Cost-Effectiveness in Health and Medicine.* New York: Oxford University Press; 1996.

# Cost – Opportunity Cost
## Accounting Cost

### BRIEF DEFINITION
Opportunity cost is the value or benefit of the best-forgone option. The opportunity cost of using a resource in a given activity is the value/benefit/return/compensation that must be forgone because the resource is not available for use in the next best option.

### EXPLANATION
The opportunity costs of using a given quantity of resources to produce a unit of health care precludes the use of those resources in their next best, most valued use. There are a number of examples that illustrate the concept of opportunity costs:

Suppose you have a certain amount of money and time to spend on a favorite pastime. The value of your money and time in their next most valuable and forgone use is the opportunity cost of the chosen pastime. Even if the pastime is free, the opportunity cost is not zero, because your time could have been spent in other valuable activities. Even though the money price of an activity may be zero, the opportunity cost is never zero as long as valuable alternatives exist.

For a health services example, the opportunity cost of the resources (ortho-pedic surgeons, anesthetists, operating room, nurses, etc) to handle traffic accidents could be the number of total hip replacements forgone per year.

Opportunity cost is the distinguishing feature between accounting costs and economic costs. Accounts have been primarily concerned with measuring costs for financial reporting purposes. **Accounting cost** is defined as historical outlay of funds that occur in the exchange or transformation of a resource. Econo-mists have been primarily concerned with measuring costs for decision-making purposes (resource allocation decisions). To achieve this objective requires that the value of the opportunities forgone be considered. The relevant costs should be explicitly measured, as the following simple algebraic relations show:

$$\text{Accounting profit} = \text{Total revenues} - \text{Accounting costs}$$
$$\text{Economic profit} = \text{Total revenues} - \text{Opportunity costs}$$

## Value and Use

Opportunity costs capture the important concept of alternative resource use. Although it is relevant in all costing, it is particularly useful when determining the cost of resources that either do not have a market price (e.g., hospital volun-teers, spouse helpers) or whose market price is hard to determine (e.g., lost patient time).

## Issues

Perhaps the biggest issue involving opportunity costs is that these costs are sometimes very difficult to measure. Cost estimates can be highly subjective and arbitrary. Nevertheless, just the recognition that opportunity costs exist for all resource use decisions is an important step toward capturing the true eco-nomic costs of scarce resource use.

## Bibliography

Call S, Holahan W. *Microeconomics.* 2nd ed. Belmont, Calif.: Wadsworth Publishing; 1983.

Drummond MF, O'Brien BJ, Stoddart GL, Torrance GW. *Methods for the Economic Evaluation of Health Care Programmes.* 2nd ed. Oxford, UK: Oxford University Press; 1997.

McGuigan JR, Moyer RC, Harris FH. *Managerial Economics: Applications, Strategy, and Tactics.* Cincinnati, Ohio: South-Western College Publishing; 1999.

# Data Coding Systems
Diagnosis-Related Group (DRG)
Major Diagnostic Category (MDC)
Strategic Product-Line Grouping
International Classification of Diseases 9th/10th Edition Clinical Modification
 (ICD 9/10 CM)
Physicians Current Procedural Terminology, Fourth Edition (CPT 4)
Health Care Cost and Utilization Project (HCUP) Coding System
National Drug Code (NDC)
Resource Intensity Weight (RIW)

## BRIEF DEFINITION
The term **data coding systems** refers to a methodology for classifying aspects of patient health and health care commonly used by health care policymakers, practitioners, and researchers to summarize the characteristics of patients and health care. This section discusses several examples of data coding systems.

## Diagnosis-Related Group (DRG)

### BRIEF DEFINITION
**Diagnosis-related group** (DRG) is a methodology for classifying patients receiving inpatient care in a hospital into a clinically homogeneous category of disease state and type of resource utilization.

### EXPLANATION
Developed at Yale University in the 1970s, DRGs were designed with the explicit objective of creating relatively homogeneous groups with respect to financial cost. Each patient's inpatient hospital stay is assigned a DRG based on principal and comorbid diagnoses, the principal and secondary procedures performed during the hospitalization, as well as the type of treatment (surgical or medical), age, sex, and discharge status.

An algorithm was developed to assign individual cases to groupings that exhibit common resource-use tendencies as measured by length of stay. Each DRG is assigned a relative weight intended to approximate the complexity and relative amount of resources used by an average case in the group. There are approximately 500 DRGs.

In 1983, the federal government, as required under the Social Security Amendments of 1983 (Public Law 98-21), initiated DRGs as the starting point in determining the amount of reimbursement to hospitals for treating Medicare patients. They are the reimbursement measures for the Prospective Payment System that began as a means to: (1) reduce the growth in Medicare outlays; (2) provide cost containment incentives to providers; and (3) maintain quality of care.

## VALUE AND USE

In the United States, Centers for Medicare and Medicaid Services (CMS, formerly the Health Care Financing Administration [HCFA]) (*see term:* Health Insurance Programs, Government – United States) uses DRGs to determine prospectively reimbursement for hospital inpatient care for Medicare beneficiaries. The amount of the prospective payment for a specific inpatient hospital stay is based on the patient's DRG. Since the provider knows the payment level per DRG beforehand, it has an incentive to identify and implement ways to deliver care as efficiently as possible, even while the patient is in the hospital.

Using DRG weights, a hospital can develop a case-mix adjusted admissions measure that can be used as a management tool for allocation of resources. Typically it is a better tool than simply the number or admissions or patient hospital days for understanding the level of resources required to serve the hospital's patient population.

In the Medicare system, the DRG payment generally covers all costs except for capital, medical education, and bad debts by Medicare patients.

## ISSUES

Although widely used, some believe DRGs do not adequately measure the complexity and severity of each patient. Additionally, the payment scheme does not seem to be consistent. Most providers believe that there is great variability in how the payment is developed—profits can be made on a small number of DRGs while other DRGs will always result in losses, no matter how much the process of care is redesigned. Moreover, there is a disincentive to have high-quality intensive care units and emergency departments in view of the fact that hospitals are paid the same amount for a particular DRG, whether or not these additional resources were used. Furthermore, DRG codes may not be very useful for health services research since some coding is subject to "DRG creep," where hospitals may choose diagnosis codes that result in higher payments, thereby maximizing their Medicare reimbursements.

## BIBLIOGRAPHY

Centers for Medicare & Medicaid Services (CMS). http://www.hcfa.gov/regs/hcfa1158p/pp021_111.doc. Accessed March 31, 2003.

Folland S, Goodman AC, Stano M. *The Economics of Health and Health Care.* Upper Saddle River, NJ: Prentice Hall; 2001.

Gapenski LC. *Understanding Health Care Financial Management.* Ann Arbor, Mich: AUPHA Press/Health Administration Press; 1983.

Jacobs P. *The Economics of Health and Medical Care.* 4th ed. Gaithersburg, Md: Aspen Publications; 1997.

## Major Diagnostic Category (MDC)

BRIEF DEFINITION

Major Diagnostic Category (MDC) refers to methodology for classifying DRGs into clinically homogeneous categories based on major body organ systems, therapeutic areas, and physician specialties.

EXPLANATION

In the United States, to effectively manage the large number of DRGs, the Centers for Medicare and Medicaid Services (*see term:* Health Insurance Programs, Government – United States) classifies each under one of 25 MDCs based on the DRGs' principal diagnosis or procedure. No DRG appears in more than one MDC. Examples include: nervous system; eye; ear, nose, mouth, and throat; respiratory system; circulatory system; digestive system; hepatobiliary system and pancreas; musculoskeletal system and connective tissue. Although the majority of MDCs correspond to a single body system or therapeutic area, some represent conditions that may impact more than one body system, such as infections or burns.

VALUE AND USE

In the past, there has not been much use for MDCs other than to use them to describe a group of DRGs. However, in the future there may be a place for MDCs as a method to determine whether health care providers should consider specializing in an area. Because providers are finding it more and more difficult to make money on many of their DRGs, a financial analysis could uncover a specialty in which the provider has low costs and good outcomes. If this were the case, a hospital could strategize to increase market share by developing the services in that MDC (recently called a "focused factory" in the literature, see Eastaugh 1998). In deciding which areas to develop, it would be difficult for a hospital to analyze the more than 500 DRGs currently used. Instead, the hospital could use the MDCs knowing that it is important to ensure a highly profitable service line, rather than using individual DRGs.

ISSUES

MDCs are not widely known or used by health providers. Although there is wide interest in grouping DRGs into functional categories, most of the literature provides methods other than the MDCs of doing so or it suggests that the process needs to be provider specific. An example of another methodology is the **strategic product-line grouping** (SPG), defined as a cluster of DRGs performed by an identified subset of the medical staff. The only difference between SPGs and MDCs is that the provider develops SPGs with extensive input from the physicians. However, both are used to determine profitability of a set of DRGs.

BIBLIOGRAPHY

Eastaugh SR. *Health Care Finance.* Gaithersburg, Md: Aspen Publications; 1998.
Jacobs P. *The Economics of Health and Medical Care.* Gaithersburg, Md: Aspen Publications; 1997.

# International Classification of Diseases 9th/10th Edition Clinical Modification (ICD 9/10 CM)

## BRIEF DEFINITION

The **International Classification of Diseases** (ICD) system is a coding system used to classify patient diagnosis as well as medical and surgical procedures.

## EXPLANATION

The Tenth Revision of the International Statistical Classification of Diseases and Related Health Problems (ICD) is the latest in a series that was formalized in 1893 as the Bertillon Classification or International List of Causes of Death. While the title has been amended to make clearer the content and purpose and to reflect the progressive extension of the scope of the classification beyond diseases and injuries, the abbreviation "ICD" has been retained. In more recent revisions, conditions have been grouped to facilitate epidemiological research and the evaluation of health care and its outcomes. Adopted in 1948 by the World Health Organization (WHO) as a basis for mortality statistics (referring to principal cause of death), this system is in its 10th edition (ICD-10), although a number of organizations have not yet migrated from the 9th edition—ICD 9 CM (www.ahima.org).

The ICD-10 system categorizes diseases into a three-character category (a single letter followed by two numbers), with one-digit and two-digit refinements or extensions. The ICD consists of more than 900 groups, which coarsely aggregate to the level of 110 main groups. The ICD 10 CM (the current version) is a two-part medical information coding system used in abstracting systems and classifying patients for DRGs. The first part consists of a comprehensive list of diseases with corresponding codes compatible with the WHO list of disease codes. The second part contains procedure codes that are independent of the disease codes.

## VALUE AND USE

ICD 9/10 CM was developed in the United States based on the WHO system and has become the standard and basis for medical care coding in the United States. Guidelines for its use as the US coding standard are published by the Centers for Medicare and Medicaid Services. The information in the medical record forms the basis of how a patient case is coded and is important in physician and hospital reimbursement, quality review, and benchmarking. Some Canadian provinces also use ICD 9 CM diagnosis and procedure codes.

## ISSUES

Because the ICD is the standard for capturing clinical data in the United States and is commonly used either directly or indirectly for reimbursement of care, many consider it appropriate for patient-level research on health care and its costs and outcomes. In this regard, studies have demonstrated its validity with certain types of claims or administrative data.

However, although code administrators strive to update codes as appropriate and eliminate ambiguities as diagnoses and health care evolve, ambiguities still may result. More troubling is misclassification of patients or care through use of codes that are partly but not entirely appropriate (e.g., to obtain a higher reimbursement level), or nonuse of codes for procedures not warranting substantial payment. These errors tend to result in suboptimal findings of the research involving data where those ICD codes are used.

BIBLIOGRAPHY

Chute CG, Cohn SP, Campbell KE, et al. The content coverage of clinical classifications. *J Am Med Inform Assoc.* 1996;3:224–233.

ICD-10 Description. http://www.who.int/whosis/icd10/descript.htm. Accessed March 31, 2003.

Jacobs P. *The Economics of Health and Medical Care.* Gaithersburg, Md: Aspen Publications; 1997.

Zweifel P. *Health Economics.* New York: Oxford Publications; 1997.

## Physicians Current Procedural Terminology, Fourth Edition (CPT 4)

### BRIEF DEFINITION

The **Physicians Current Procedural Terminology** (CPT) system is a listing developed by the American Medical Association (AMA) of descriptive terms and identifying codes that describe medical, surgical, and diagnostic services.

### EXPLANATION

The purpose of CPT is to provide a uniform language and therefore an effective means for reliable nationwide communication among physicians, patients, and payers. Each CPT code contains five numeric digits for billable medical procedures.

The AMA first developed and published CPT in 1966. The first edition helped encourage the use of standard terms and descriptors to document procedures in the medical record; helped communicate accurate information on procedures and services to agencies concerned with insurance claims; provided the basis for a computer-oriented system to evaluate operative procedures; and contributed basic information for actuarial and statistical purposes.

The fourth edition, published in 1977, represented significant updates in medical technology and introduced a procedure of periodic updating to keep pace with the rapidly changing medical environment. In 1983, the CPT code was adopted as part of the Health Care Financing Administration's (HCFA) health care common procedure coding system. In July 1987, as part of the Omnibus Budget Reconciliation Act, HCFA (now CMS) mandated the use of CPT for reporting outpatient hospital surgical procedures.

In 1992, Medicare revised its payments to physicians based on a resource-based relative value scale approach. At the same time, to ensure more consistent coding by physicians, the AMA adopted significant changes in how physicians' evaluation and management services were defined under the CPT methodology. The AMA also introduced guidelines for coding these services, including the extent of history taking and physical examination. When implemented, there was a shift toward higher reimbursement for primary care physicians. The CPT guidelines for evaluation and management were further refined in 1998. Each year an updated version is prepared. The most recent version, CPT-2002, contains 8,107 codes and descriptors.

VALUE AND USE

CPT codes were developed for reporting reimbursable medical services and procedures used by physicians, primarily in the outpatient setting. Most of the inpatient medical services are billed by the hospital using the ICD system. Interestingly, the CPT system makes no pretense regarding comprehensiveness, particularly because the CPT codes are only widely used for outpatient procedures.

The CPT terminology is the most widely accepted medical nomenclature used to report medical procedures and services under public and private health insurance programs. CPT is also used for administrative management purposes such as claims processing and developing guidelines for medical care review. The uniform language is likewise applicable to medical education and research by providing a useful basis for local, regional, and national utilization comparisons.

ISSUES

Although more responsive and not as cumbersome to understand as the ICD system, the CPT methodology still causes confusion for some. It appears that many family physicians find it difficult to classify certain visits and that some physicians have not fully learned the definitions and guidelines of the current coding system. Additionally, because CPT codes are designed to capture procedures, not treatments, some physicians are confused as to how to code certain treatments.

BIBLIOGRAPHY

AMA Web site. http://www.ama-assn.org/ama/pub/category/3882.html. Accessed June 1, 2001.
Chute CG, Cohn SP, Campbell KE, et al. The content coverage of clinical classifications. *J Am Med Inform Assoc.* 1996;3:224–233.
Yao P, Wiggs BR, Gregor C, et al. Discordance between physicians and coders in assignment of diagnoses. *Int J Qual Health.* 1999;11:147–153.

# Health Care Cost and Utilization Project (HCUP) Coding System

BRIEF DEFINITION

The **Health Care Cost and Utilization Project (HCUP) Coding System** classifies hospital outpatients and physicians' office services for reimbursement under Medicare and some state Medicaid programs (*see term:* Health Insurance Programs, Government – United States).

EXPLANATION

The HCUP Coding System was developed by the Health Care Financing Administration (HCFA, currently the Centers for Medicare and Medicaid Services [CMS]) and is used to classify services provided in the hospital outpatient and physicians' office settings that are covered under Medicare and many state Medicaid programs (administered and/or funded by Medicare). It is divided into three levels: Level I consists of CPT-4 codes for physician services; Level II consists of national codes for medical services, products, and supplies (including durable medical equipment) not included in Level I; Level III consists of local codes for services. The HCUP National Panel establishes the Level II alphanumeric HCUP procedure and modifier codes, their long and short descriptions, and applicable Medicare administrative, coverage, and pricing data. All CPT codes are HCUP codes but not all HCUP codes are CPT codes. National codes are updated annually.

VALUE AND USE

CMS mandates the use of the HCUP Coding System to report services for Part B of the Medicare Program. In October 1986, CMS also required state Medicaid agencies to use HCUP codes in the Medicaid Management Information System.

ISSUES

HCUP codes were selected for use in HIPAA transactions, which will very likely increase their importance to providers and to health services researchers.

BIBLIOGRAPHY

HCFA Web site. http://www.cms.gov/medicare/hcpcs. Accessed September 20, 2003.

## National Drug Code (NDC)

BRIEF DEFINITION

The **National Drug Code** (NDC) is the numeric name or code assigned to each pharmaceutical product.

EXPLANATION

The US Food and Drug Administration (FDA) developed the NDC, and each drug receives its unique code or codes once approved by the FDA. A drug has unique codes for different doses and package sizes. The NDC was initially established as an essential part of an out-of-hospital drug reimbursement program under Medicare.

The NDC was developed as a result of the Drug Listing Act of 1972, which made available to the commissioner of the FDA a current list of all drugs manufactured, prepared, processed, or sold by a drug manufacturer registered under the Federal Food, Drug, and Cosmetic Act. This act requires submission of information on commercially marketed drugs.

Each drug dose and package is assigned a unique 10-digit, three-segment number that identifies the labeler/vendor, product, and package size. The NDC has a hierarchy of 21 major and 139 minor drug classifications, and is updated quarterly within five working days after the end of March, June, September, and December.

VALUE AND USE

The NDC facilitates drug reimbursement to retail pharmacists and Medicaid programs among others. The NDC was intended to provide a standard way of identifying drug products, and it now serves as a universal identifier for prescription drugs and a few selected over-the-counter drugs.

ISSUES

Overall, there do not seem to be issues in the development of codes or use of the NDC. The hierarchy of code levels is one way in which the FDA makes the NDC useful to clinicians and researchers. Another way is by allowing the pharmaceutical firm to assign the second and third segments of the code.

BIBLIOGRAPHY

FDA Web site. http://www.fda.gov/cder/ndc/index.htm. Accessed September 20, 2003.

Gu H, Liu L, Halper M, et al. Converting an integrated hospital formulary into an object-oriented database representation. *Proc AMIA Annu Fall Symp.* 1998;770–774.

## Resource Intensity Weight (RIW)

BRIEF DEFINITION

**Resource Intensity Weight** (RIW) estimates the relative resources used by patients receiving inpatient hospital care (inpatients) and those undergoing outpatient surgical procedures (day surgery patients).

EXPLANATION

RIWs are ratios that measure expected use of resources and are registered trademarks of the Canadian Institute for Health Information (CIHI, formerly the Hospital Medical Records Institute ). A schedule of RIWs is developed and published annually by CIHI based on its case mix group (CMG) grouper, which is similar to DRGs in the United States, for inpatients and on its Comprehensive Ambulatory Classification system (CACS) for ambulatory care patients. These weights were previously based on US charge data (1985 New York data for 1991 grouper; 1991/92 Maryland data for 1993 grouper) in combination with Canadian data provided by the Ontario Case Costing Project. As of 2000, primarily Canadian data are being used because US practice patterns and associated costs were not representative of Canadian care and costs.

An example of a typical calculation (in 1995 dollars) is detailed here:

For stroke, the New York State Service Intensity Weight (NYSI) is \$3900.63, the CIHI average length of stay is 15 days, and the New York average length of stay is 13.9 days. Therefore the New York routine cost per day is \$271.61, and the standardized relative cost for the entire CIHI database is \$1561.84. The RIW for stroke = typical cost/1561.84. Typical cost is computed by adding 3900.63 to the product of (15 − 13.9) and 271.61. The result is a RIW of 2.68.

By using data from New York and Canada, the RIW attempts to adjust for the differences that exist. The result is interpreted as a stroke case that is estimated to use 2.68 times as many resources as the average typical case in the CIHI database.

RIWs were developed responding to the need of Ontario health providers (as expressed to the CIHI) for a measure of hospital output that would be fairer and more flexible than the measures instituted in Canada in the early 1970s as a part of global hospital budgets.

### VALUE AND USE

Canadian hospitals use CMGs together with RIWs (which define the financial dimension of each patient) to provide data concerning the relationship between clinical and financial data in utilization management. It is important in Canada to understand this tool to plan, manage, and be reimbursed for medical services. RIWs were developed in 1989 and first used in 1990 to determine growth and equity funding of Ontario hospitals. Much of Canada now uses RIWs to adjust payments to hospitals, prepare budgets, and allocate resources within a hospital.

### ISSUES

Although these tools are rarely used outside Canada, RIWs mirror other countries' attempts to categorize patients and their care. For example, in the United States, the DRG and resource-based relative value systems are used.

Additionally, cost estimates and RIWs for the patients in each case mix group should be calculated from a representative Canadian database of patient-specific costs. Currently, Ontario costs are being used as reflective of national Canadian costs. Shortly, RIWs will only encompass Canadian data.

### BIBLIOGRAPHY

Benoit D, Skea W, Mitchell S. Developing cost weights with limited cost data—experiences using Canadian cost data. *Casemix Quarterly.* 2000;2:88–96.

Case Mix Groups (CMJ) Overview. http://www.umanitoba.ca/centres/mchp/concept/dict/CMG_overview.html. Accessed March 31, 2003.

*Casemix Quarterly.* http://www.casemix.org. Accessed March 31, 2003.

Pink GH, Bolley HB. Physicians in health care management: 3. Case mix groups and resource intensity weights: An overview for physicians. *Can Med Assoc J.* 1994;150:889–894.

Pink GH, Hildo B. Physicians in health care management: 4. Case mix groups and resource intensity weights: Physicians and hospital funding. *Can Med Assoc J.* 1994;150:1255–1261.

# Decision Analysis
## Expectation

### BRIEF DEFINITION
**Decision analysis** is a quantitative approach to decision making under uncertainty in which all relevant elements of the decision—alternative actions, chance events (along with their probabilities of occurrence), and final consequences—are stated explicitly in a model. This model typically takes the form of either a decision tree or an influence diagram and permits the decision maker to determine systematically the relative value of alternative courses of action.

### EXPLANATION
Decision analysis provides a framework for decision making based upon an explicit structure that illustrates what is known, what is uncertain, what can be done, what the likely outcomes are, and which decisions yield the most favorable outcomes. In conducting decision analysis, the modeling (*see term:* Modeling) process can illustrate the entire "structure" of the decision, thereby improving understanding of the important issues. Given agreement on the overall structure of the decision model, the analysis can help inform the decision maker as to which alternative decision yields the most favorable outcome under the given circumstances. Decision analysis does not predict what consequence a specific decision will have in a particular case, but can answer complicated questions such as "which is the least risky alternative?"

There are six basic steps in the structuring of a decision analysis:

1. Statement of the problem and identification of the decision maker whose perspective is being taken.
2. Enumeration of alternative courses of action and the possible consequences of each action.
3. Statement of the standard by which outcomes will be valued and alternatives compared. This is typically phrased as an objective or set of objectives (e.g., costs, health benefits, profit) to be optimized.
4. Modeling of the decision:
   - Elaboration of a model of the decision structure (perhaps using a decision tree or an influence diagram)
   - Specification of the consequences of each alternative decision choice and the probabilities of those consequences or "events"
   - Assignment of values (e.g., cost and/or utility) to each final outcome, incorporating the decision maker's preferences
5. Identification of the best alternative or alternatives.
6. Sensitivity analysis.

Identification of the preferred decision, and perhaps a "recommendation to decision makers" can be made by comparing each alternative's expected value, or **expectation**—the weighted average of all possible consequences, based on the probabilities of the events that follow a decision. Sensitivity analysis (*see term:* Sensitivity Analysis) examines the changes in expected values and recommendations when the values of uncertain or unknown parameters are varied.

## VALUE AND USE

Decision analysis provides a formal and rational approach to making decisions, one that allows key structural and input assumptions to be made transparent, explicit, and even visual. It is an analytical tool that can inform decision makers as to which decision(s) will yield optimal results. This in turn can help in the formulation of better policies.

Of course, a decision analysis can illustrate the dominance of one strategy over another if it exists. More typically, especially in complex decision-making environments like health care research and clinical medicine, the steps required to build a model that accurately represents a decision can help uncover crucial assumptions and relationships (e.g., between practice patterns, clinical outcomes, and economic costs) that may not be readily understood by clinicians or decision makers either because of such factors as traditional practices or significant separation in time between cause and effect. Sensitivity analysis can guide further research by highlighting key uncertainties that seem to have the greatest impact on identification of a strategy as optimal.

Decision analysis provides the conceptual foundation for cost-effectiveness analysis (*see term:* Cost-Effectiveness Analysis), which can be used to inform decisions regarding the allocation of scarce health care resources.

## ISSUES

The prescriptions offered by decision analysis are only valid to the extent that the model structure adequately represents the true process and that the values given to model parameters are accurate. Decision analysis does not guarantee good outcomes, but it is a systematic method of making the best decisions using the available data. At the least, decision analysis identifies those model structural aspects or parameters where data are missing or scarce.

The focus is on helping people make more informed choices rather than determining those choices. In that spirit, it is useful to bear in mind the distinction between good decisions and good outcomes. Decision analysis aims to promote a more reasoned, formal approach to the process of decision making.

## BIBLIOGRAPHY

Holloway CA. *Decision Making Under Uncertainty: Models and Choices.* Englewood Cliffs, NJ: Prentice-Hall; 1979.

Hunink M, Glasziou P, et al. *Decision Making in Health and Medicine.* Cambridge, UK: Cambridge University Press; 2001.

Raiffa H. *Decision Analysis.* Reading, Mass: Addison-Wesley Publishing; 1968.

Weinstein MC, Fineberg HV, et al. *Clinical Decision Analysis.* Philadelphia: W.B. Saunders, 1980.

# Decision Tree
Decision Nodes
Chance Nodes
Pathway Outcomes

## BRIEF DEFINITION

A **decision tree** is a flow diagram depicting the logical structure of a choice under conditions of uncertainty, including all relevant alternative decisions available to the decision maker as well as the values and probabilities of all relevant downstream consequences (*see term:* Modeling).

## EXPLANATION

A decision tree is a graphical representation of a decision maker's options and their likely consequences (an example is shown in Figure 1). It contains four basic elements:

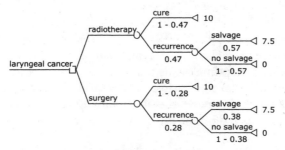

Figure 1.  Example of a decision tree
From Roest FHJ, et al. *Medical Decision Making.* Vol. 17,
pp. 285–291. Copyright © 1997 by Medical Decision Making.
Reprinted by permission of Sage Publications, Inc.

1. **Decision nodes** indicate instances where the decision maker has a choice of one or more possible courses of action. Branches leading out of a given decision node represent different choices.

2. **Chance nodes** indicate uncertain outcomes beyond the control of the decision maker. Branches leading out of a given chance node represent mutually exclusive, collectively exhaustive, and probabilistically determined events.

3. Each chance node is assigned a probability to represent the likelihood of the events emerging from a chance node.

4. **Pathway outcomes** (or payoffs), denominated in units of the decision maker's objective and assigned to the terminal end of each branch of the decision tree, are assigned to each possible combination of choice and chance.

The optimal decision is computed via a process called "folding back" (see Figure 2):

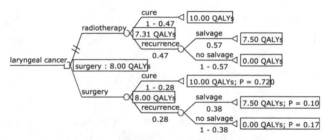

Figure 2. Computation of an optimal decision
From Roest FHJ, et al. *Medical Decision Making.* Vol. 17,
pp. 285–291. Copyright © 1997 by Medical Decision Making.
Reprinted by permission of Sage Publications, Inc.

1. Beginning at the ends of the decision tree, expected values are computed for each chance node by multiplying pathway outcomes by their probabilities. This is commonly referred to as "averaging out."

2. At each decision node, a single action is chosen that produces the most favorable outcome value. All other actions are eliminated from consideration. This is commonly referred to as "folding back."

3. The process of averaging out and folding back assigns to every node in the decision tree the optimal value that can be attained at any time the decision maker is at that node. Most importantly, it assigns the optimal value to the initial decision node, thereby highlighting the course of action that seems optimal based on the information presented in the tree.

## VALUE AND USE

Decision trees provide a relatively simple means of organizing and communicating the elements of a decision analysis.

Decision trees are useful in pharmacoeconomics by providing a methodologically transparent structure with which to determine cost of care in a given disease or disorder, as well as the cost-effectiveness of alternative therapies. Decision trees can also be used to enable clinicians, researchers, and decision makers to better understand where data are missing or scarce in determining the cost of care or cost-effectiveness of alternatives. In those cases in which the data are reasonably comprehensive and accurate, the value of the decision tree is maximized. Inputs into the tree may include published data from clinical trials, epidemiology studies, and observational studies or, when those are limited, the input from clinical experts.

## ISSUES

While decision trees can convey a great deal of detail about the structure and data underlying a decision-analytic problem, they can quickly grow to a size that is either unmanageable for the modeler, uninterpretable by the reviewer, or both. Thus, decision models that are clinically complete may be overly complicated to construct or to interpret. Consequently, researchers trying to communicate the key structural elements of a choice under conditions of uncertainty may choose to supplement or complement their efforts with alternative graphical representations (e.g., influence diagram [*see term:* Influence Diagram] or state-transition model [*see term:* Modeling]). For example, a model of the treatment of a chronic disease may require a long period of time to sufficiently unfold, or it may require dividing the problem's time perspective into many fine intervals to capture relevant events. Markov modeling techniques can be used in such cases, often as a part of a decision tree.

Other specific issues relate to the data inputs that are important in formulating the ultimate results of analyses using decision trees. First, the probability data for certain chance outcomes may be lacking in the literature, especially if those outcomes are relatively rare events that can be highly significant if costs are being considered. Second, if clinical literature is used in developing probability values, errors may result because of variability in clinical outcomes and because the true population value is unknown. Third, the impact of outlier patients which are often seen in clinical trials can have a significant effect on terminal outcomes, especially costs, and it is difficult to determine if these patients are true outliers or whether they are really present at that level in the population.

BIBLIOGRAPHY

Detsky AS, Naglie G, Krahn MD, et al. Primer on decision analysis: Part 1—getting started. *Med Decis Making.* 1997;17:123–125.

Hunink M, Glasziou P, et al. *Decision Making in Health and Medicine.* Cambridge, UK: Cambridge University Press; 2001.

Weinstein, MC, Fineberg HV, et al. *Clinical Decision Analysis.* Philadelphia: W.B. Saunders; 1980.

# Delphi Panel Method

## BRIEF DEFINITION

The **Delphi Panel Method** is a structured method of eliciting expert judgment that is particularly useful as a tool to achieve consensus of opinion when the decisive factors are subjective and not knowledge-based.

## EXPLANATION

Delphi is a method for structuring a group communication process to allow a group of individuals to deal with complex problems. It consists of a series of interrogations in which the anonymous responses of group members are submitted to the group for comment until consensus, divergence, or stasis of opinion is reached.

The Delphi Panel Method generally follows the following procedural outline:

1. The problem is identified.
2. An expert panel is developed.

3. The panel is presented the problem and asked to respond.
4. Responses are synthesized into a series of statements.
5. The synthesized statements are submitted to the panel.
6. The panel responds.
7. The process continues until convergence, divergence, or stasis is identified.

Delphi studies typically share three distinctive features: anonymity of response, feedback of individual responses to the group, and statistical analyses using median and dispersion.

## VALUE AND USE

The Delphi Panel Method is a useful technique to derive parameter estimates for data elements whose values are not known. This method can prove useful for estimating data regarding effectiveness and appropriateness estimation, as well as in determining appropriate estimates for unknown clinical or economic parameters.

The Delphi method was designed to optimize the use of group opinion while minimizing the adverse qualities of interacting groups, such as dominance by influential participants and unwillingness to participate fully in group decision situations.

## ISSUES

A number of issues regarding the Delphi Panel Method have been documented in the literature. Most commonly, the Delphi method is criticized for its lack of adherence to traditional statistical comparisons. In addition, it can be difficult to evaluate fully the accuracy and reliability of this method since the opinions of panel members may be person- and situation-specific. Because of this, it is difficult to compare subsequent applications of the methodology to previous work. Another consideration is that the composition of the panel must be carefully considered in order to help ensure appropriate study outcomes.

Because of these limitations, many have suggested the Delphi Panel Method be a method of last resort to deal with complex problems where no other models exist. In these circumstances, the Delphi Panel Method may provide useful information that does not exist otherwise.

## BIBLIOGRAPHY

Jones J, Hunter D. Qualitative research: Consensus methods for medical and health services research. *BMJ.* 1995;311:376–380.

Lang T. An overview of four futures methodologies (delphi, environmental scanning, issues management and emerging issue analysis). *Manoa J.* 1995;7:1–43.

Linstone HA, Turoff M. *The Delphi Method: Techniques and Applications.* Reading, Mass: Addison-Wesley; 1975.

Twining J. *A Naturalistic Inquiry into the Collaboratory: In Search of Understanding for Prospective Participants* [PhD dissertation]. Denton: Texas Woman's University School of Library and Information Studies; 1999.

# Disability-Adjusted Life Year (DALY)

## BRIEF DEFINITION

**Disability-adjusted life year** (DALY) can be defined as a unit of measurement of the impact of disease in terms of both time lost due to premature death (mortality) and time lived with a disability (morbidity).

## EXPANDED DEFINITION

The Global Burden of Disease Study (GBD), sponsored by the World Bank, was initiated in 1992 with the aim of quantifying the burden of disease and injury on human populations. Such a quantification required a unit of measurement that considered both mortality and morbidity. For this reason the concept of DALY was developed.

The total impact of a disease is not only the loss of life resulting from premature mortality but also the disability, impairment, pain, and misery—collectively known as morbidity. For example, let us take a hypothetical situation of a woman who sustained a hip fracture at the age of 58 years, suffered for the next

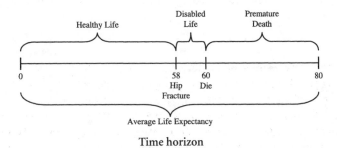

Time horizon

two years, and died at the age of 60 (see figure). This woman not only lost 20 years of her life (assuming an average life expectancy of 80 years for a female), but also spent two years of her life with disability because of hip fracture.

For the calculation of a DALY, the impact of a particular disease on mortality is estimated using the difference between the average life expectancy and the age at which death occurred and is expressed as years of life lost (YLL). Because average life expectancies vary by country, the method is standardized by using the average life expectancy data from the country with the highest figures (Japan).

$$YLL_i = \text{Average Life Expectancy} - \text{Age at Death}_i,$$

where $YLL_i$ = the years of life lost by the $i$th individual, and Age at Death$_i$ = age at death for the $i$th individual.

For the impact of morbidity on the DALY, years lived with disability (YLD) is measured by considering the following factors: the extent of disability associated with different nonfatal conditions (disability weights), the relative importance of healthy life at different ages (age weights), and the time preference for health which is the value of health gained now as compared to the value of health gained in the future. Thus,

$$DALY_i = YLL_i + YLD_i,$$

where $DALY_i$ = DALY of the ith individual and $YLD_i$ = YLD of the ith individual.

DALYs of different individuals can be summed to estimate the total DALYs in a country and then summed across nations to estimate the global DALYs.

The quality-adjusted life year (QALY) (*see term:* Quality-Adjusted Life Year [QALY]) is another commonly used unit of measurement for health. The QALY, however, differs in three important ways from the DALY:

1. The life expectancy used in the QALY is situation-specific. For example, the QALYs gained from an intervention tested in clinical trial would compare the mortality experience of the treatment group to that of the control group. The life expectancy used in the DALY is based on an external standard (Japan).

2. The disability weights in the QALY are based on preferences (e.g., utilities), either measured on the general public or on the patients in the trial. Moreover, the preferences are on a continuous scale from 0 to 1. The disability weights in the DALY are not utilities, but are person trade-off scores from a panel of health care workers, and the scores are on a discrete scale with only seven categories.

3. The QALY does not use age weights. The DALY uses age weights that give lower weight to years of the young and the elderly.

## Value and Use

The DALY captures the impact of both morbidity and mortality in a common unit of measurement. Therefore, DALY may be used to facilitate epidemiological surveillance of the total disease burden across disease categories and over time (i.e., number of DALYs). It has been suggested that the DALY, being a common measurement unit, would be particularly useful when conducting cost-effectiveness analyses of different interventions or treatments for chronic diseases or disabling health conditions (i.e., cost per DALY avoided). The proponents of the DALY approach have also suggested that DALYs could provide policymakers with the information needed for identifying the optimal package of health care services deliverable within a fixed budget. However, the usefulness of DALYs for cost-effectiveness analyses and health care resource allocation is still under debate.

## Issues

Since its introduction in 1993, the DALY approach of quantifying disease burden has been debated heavily, and many have questioned its validity and the underlying value judgment. Many researchers have argued that the preference weights applied in the DALY approach were only based on the preferences of the expert panel, which might not represent the preferences of society as a whole. QALYs, on the other hand, are usually derived using societal preference weights (e.g., EQ-5D). The DALY approach has also been criticized for violating the principle of treating all people equally. The reason for this criticism is that the inclusion of unequal age weights in the DALY may introduce a bias against both children (who have little disability compared to the aged) and the elderly (who have shorter survival compared to younger individuals). In addition to concerns with the age weights, the inclusion of disability weights has also been controversial in that such weights may presume that the life years of disabled individuals are worth less than the life years of individuals without disabilities. Therefore, the validity and equity of resource allocation decisions made using the DALY approach have been questioned by some.

In response, the World Health Organization (WHO) has promised to address these controversies in later versions of the Global Burden of Disease studies. Despite its limitations, the DALY approach provides a reasonable means to measure the burden of disease in a population.

BIBLIOGRAPHY

Anand S, Hanson K. Disability-adjusted life years: a critical review. *J Health Econ.* 1997;16:685–702.

Arnesen T, Nord E. The value of DALY life: problems with ethics and validity of disability adjusted life years. *BMJ.* 1999;319:1423–1425.

Murray CJL, Lopez AD, eds. The global burden of disease: a comprehensive assessment of mortality and disability from diseases, injuries and risk factors in 1990 and projected to 2020. Cambridge, Mass: Harvard School of Public Health on behalf of the World Health Organization and the World Bank (Global Burden of Disease and Injury Series, Vol. I); 1996.

# Discounting
## Discount Rate

### BRIEF DEFINITION
**Discounting** is a method used to adjust future costs and benefits to their present market value.

### EXPLANATION
If we had the choice to receive something of value (e.g., a new car) today versus sometime in the future, we would prefer to receive it today. Our preference to consume today versus tomorrow means that things of value (e.g., costs and benefits of health care interventions) are worth less if they occur in the future than if they occur today. To be able to consider future costs and benefits in decision making today, we must adjust future values to reflect their present day value. This procedure is referred to as discounting. The **discount rate** is the rate at which future costs and benefits are adjusted to reflect their present value.

## VALUE AND USE

Because discounting involves converting future value into present value, a commonly used formula for discounting is as follows:

Where interest rate $= r$, the value of $1 received $n$ years from now is $1/(1 + r)^n$.

For example, let us say that one has an opportunity to purchase several cases of vintage wines for $10000. It is known that the cases of wines will sell for $11000 one year from now. Would it make sense to invest $10000 that will fetch $11000 one year from today? To evaluate the current value of $11000 one year from now (assuming an 8% interest rate), we will use our discounting formula.

$$\text{Current value} = 11000/(1 + 0.08)^1 = \$10185.19$$

The present value of the wine that will sell for $11000 one year from today is $10185.19. Since the present value of the future revenue is greater than the present cost, it makes sense to invest in the wines.

## ISSUES

When carrying out an economic analysis, selecting the discount rate is of great concern. The general consensus rule is to discount either at 3% or 5% and carry out a sensitivity analysis between 0% and 10%. The majority opinion is that costs and benefits should be discounted at the same rate; however, there are some pharmacoeconomic experts who feel that outcomes should be discounted at a different rate or should not be discounted at all.

## BIBLIOGRAPHY

Boardman AE, Greenberg DH, Vining AR, Weimer DL. Benefits and costs in different time periods: the mechanics of discounting. In: *Cost Benefit Analysis Concepts and Practices.* Upper Saddle River, NJ: Prentice-Hall; 1996.

Bootman JL, Townsend RJ, McGhan WF. Cost determination and analysis. In: *Principles of Pharmacoeconomics.* Cincinnati, Ohio: Harvey Whitney Books Company; 1996.

Mullins CD, Merchant S. Guidelines and information requirements. In: Zollo S, ed. *Introduction to Applied Pharmacoeconomics.* New York: McGraw-Hill Companies, Inc; 2001.

# Disease Management

## Disease Management Support Services

### BRIEF DEFINITION

**Disease management** is a system of coordinated health care interventions and communications for populations with conditions in which patient self-care efforts are significant.

### EXPLANATION

Disease management is an evolving concept in health care delivery that seeks to improve clinical outcomes while reducing total system-wide health care costs. Disease management (DM) is a patient-focused, comprehensive approach that seeks to improve the patient's clinical, economic, and humanistic outcomes. Disease management:

- Supports the physician or practitioner/patient relationship and plan of care,
- Emphasizes prevention of exacerbations and complications using evidence-based practice guidelines and patient empowerment strategies, and
- Evaluates clinical, humanistic, and economic outcomes on an ongoing basis with the goal of improving overall health.

Disease management programs include all six of the following elements, while programs consisting of fewer components are **disease management support services**. Disease management components include

- Population identification processes
- Evidence-based practice guidelines
- Collaborative practice models to include physician and support-service providers
- Patient self-management education (which may include primary prevention, behavior modification programs, and compliance/surveillance)
- Process and outcomes measurement, evaluation, and management
- Routine reporting/feedback loop (which may include communication with patient, physician, health plan, and ancillary providers, and practice profiling)

## VALUE AND USE

Disease management programs reflect the confluence and application of public health services, clinical practice guidelines, evidence-based medicine, and outcomes research concepts. Disease management initiatives provide an excellent opportunity to understand the value of pharmaceutical products in the clinical, humanistic, and economic outcomes of patient treatment in a naturalistic environment.

## ISSUES

Comprehensive disease management programs require collaboration among many health care providers; however, it is consequently difficult to create incentives for all health care providers to provide more efficient use of health care resources.

Not all medical conditions are candidates for disease management, and not all programs produce favorable results.

While many health systems have begun to implement disease management programs, the acceptance and use of disease management programs may not satisfy all organizational objectives (e.g., clinical and financial).

## BIBLIOGRAPHY

Disease Management Association of America. http://www.dmaa.org/definition.html. Accessed January 2003.

Navarro RP, Christensen D, Leider H. *Disease Management Programs in Managed Care Pharmacy Practice.* Gaithersburg, Md: Aspen Publications; 1999.

# Dominance
Simple Dominance
Extended Dominance
Efficient Frontier

BRIEF DEFINITION

**Dominance** refers to a situation in which one alternative is dominated by another, and accordingly the dominated alternative should be ruled out of contention. There are two ways an alternative can be dominated: **simple dominance** and **extended dominance**. In simple dominance, there is another alternative that is both more effective and less costly (*see term:* Cost-Effectiveness Analysis). In extended dominance, there is another alternative that is more effective and more costly, but provides better value for money. When all dominated alternatives are eliminated, the remaining terms form the **efficient frontier**.

EXPLANATION

Simple dominance is also known as "strong dominance." Extended dominance is also known as "weak dominance." Extended dominance can occur only if there are three or more alternatives, although this can include the do-nothing alternative.

Dominance is explained below using an example adapted from Hunink and colleagues (2001). There are seven alternative programs, including the do-nothing alternative, only one of which can be implemented, in the table. All costs of each program have been comprehensively computed relative to the do-nothing alternative and are shown in dollars. All outcomes of each program have also been comprehensively determined and are shown as the number of quality-adjusted life years (QALYs) (*see term:* Quality-Adjusted Life Year [QALY]) gained relative to the do-nothing alternative. The programs are listed in order of increasing cost.

First, programs that are dominated by simple dominance are eliminated. P2 is dominated by P1 because it is both more costly and less effective. Similarly, P6 is dominated by P5. P2 and P6 are thus ruled out of contention and this is indicated by "dominated" in the Incremental Cost-Effectiveness Ratio (ICER) columns.

Second, the initial incremental cost-effectiveness ratios (column 4) (*see term:* Cost-Effectiveness Analysis) are calculated by comparing each program to the one above it in the table ignoring the dominated programs. If there is no extended dominance, these numbers will be nondecreasing. That is, each number will be equal to or greater than the number above it. We see in this table that this is not so. P4 has an ICER of 60000 while P5 has only 15000. This indicates that P4 is dominated by P5 using extended dominance. The reason is that it would never be sensible from a cost-effectiveness point of view to implement P4, given that we have P5 available. If we were willing to implement P4, we are saying we would be willing to pay $60000 per QALY. In that case, we should definitely implement P5 because we can purchase the additional QALYs for

Comparison of the Cost-Effectiveness of Sample Programs

| (1) | (2) | | (3) | | (4) | (5) |
|---|---|---|---|---|---|---|
| | | Effectiveness (E) (number of QALYs) | Incremental Cost ($\Delta C$) | Incremental Effectiveness ($\Delta E$) | Initial Incremental Cost-Effectiveness Ratio ($\Delta C/\Delta E$) | Final Incremental Cost-Effectiveness Ratio ($\Delta C/\Delta E$) |
| Program | Cost (C) ($) | | | | | |
| P0 (do nothing) | 0 | 0 | — | — | — | — |
| P1 | 100000 | 20 | 100000 | 20 | 5000 | 5000 |
| P2 | 220000 | 18 | — | — | Dominated | Dominated |
| P3 | 420000 | 36 | 320000 | 16 | 20000 | 20000 |
| P4 | 540000 | 38 | 120000 | 2 | 60000 | Dominated (extended) |
| P5 | 660000 | 46 | 120000 | 8 | 15000 | — |
| | | | 240000 | 10 | — | 24000 |
| P6 | 720000 | 44 | — | — | Dominated | Dominated |

only \$15000 each. Thus, P4 is ruled out by extended dominance, and this is indicated in column 5.

Third, the final and correct ICER results are computed in column 5 by comparing each program to the one above it in the table, ignoring all dominated alternatives. These are the correct ratios and those that should be used in presenting the cost-effectiveness results. The interpretation of this example is that if the decision threshold for cost per QALY was equal to or greater than \$5000 but less than \$20000, P1 should be implemented. If it was equal to or greater than \$20000 but less than \$24000, P3 should be implemented; and if it was equal to or greater than \$24000, P5 should be implemented. P1, P3, and P5 are said to form the efficient frontier because all are efficient in the sense of not being dominated and the decision among them is simply based on the decision maker's threshold cost per QALY.

Dominance is a tricky concept, and readers who want more details should consult the teaching references listed in the Bibliography.

## VALUE AND USE

Dominance is a technical concept that is crucial to the correct interpretation of cost-effectiveness and cost-utility results.

The reason for identifying and removing dominated alternatives is economic. Since the goal of a cost-effectiveness analysis is to determine which treatment options produce more effect for the cost, it makes sense to remove options that clearly cost more but are less effective. Checking alternatives for simple dominance is one way to remove options that will not promote cost-effectiveness. Similarly, removing options dominated by extended dominance removes options that do not provide good incremental value for money compared to an available alternative.

In cost-effectiveness and cost-utility articles and reports, it is customary to list all of the alternatives and indicate those that were dominated in the ICER column. It is understood that options labeled "dominated" were excluded from further analysis.

If only two alternatives are being compared and one is more effective but costs less, there is no need to conduct an analysis. Simply choose the dominant alternative.

ISSUES

Dominance is a complex technical concept. Unfortunately, it is often poorly understood and poorly handled in analyses, particularly extended dominance. In critically appraising studies, readers should pay careful attention to whether dominance has been handled correctly or not.

Simple dominance is uncontroversial and always appropriate. Extended dominance, however, is more complicated because of possible budget implications. If, for example, there is sufficient budget for P4 but insufficient for P5, should P4 be implemented? Or alternatively, should P5 be implemented but on a scaled-down basis? If so, does the scaled-down version of P5 have the same incremental cost-effectiveness as the full version? Or, alternatively, should a budget increase be sought, or should funds be diverted from other less cost-effective programs? These are the real issues that the decision makers must deal with. Nevertheless, the use of extended dominance still gives the best guidance on maximizing value for money.

BIBLIOGRAPHY

Drummond MF, O'Brien BJ, Stoddart GL, Torrance GW. *Methods for the Economic Evaluation of Health Care Programmes.* 2nd ed. Oxford, UK: Oxford University Press; 1997.

Hunink M, Glasziou P, Siegel J, et al. *Decision-Making in Health and Medicine: Integrating Evidence and Values.* Cambridge, UK: Cambridge University Press; 2001.

Seigel JE, Weinstein MC, Torrance GW. Reporting Cost-Effectiveness Studies and Results. In: Gold MR, Siegel JE, Russell LB, Weinstein MC, eds. *Cost-effectiveness in Health and Medicine.* New York: Oxford University Press; 1996.

# Drug

| | |
|---|---|
| Synthetic Drug | Effective Patent Life |
| Biologic | Line Extension |
| Prescription Drug | Generic Drug |
| Over-the-Counter Drug | Me-Too Drug |
| Ethical Drug | Multiple Source Drug |

BRIEF DEFINITION

A **drug** is defined as any chemical compound that may be used as an aid in the diagnosis, treatment, or prevention of disease or other clinical condition. Drugs are administered for the relief of pain or suffering, or to control or improve any physiologic or pathologic condition.

EXPLANATION

The above definition could also be used as the definition of a medicine or remedy and could apply to food supplements such as vitamins and minerals. In the United States, in practical usage, the term "drug" is limited to those substances that are regulated by the US Food and Drug Administration (FDA) (*see term:* Food and Drug Administration [FDA]). In the United States, the Food, Drug, and Cosmetic Act (Code of Federal Regulations Title 21) defines drugs as follows.

The term "drug" means
(A) articles recognized in the official United States Pharmacopoeia, the official Homoeopathic Pharmacopoeia of the United States, or official National Formulary, or any supplement to any of them; and

(B) articles intended for use in the diagnosis, cure, mitigation, treatment, or prevention of disease in man or other animals; and

(C) articles (other than food) intended to affect the structure or any function of the body of man or other animals; and

(D) articles intended for use as a component of any article specified in clause (A), (B), or (C). A food or dietary supplement for which a claim, subject to sections 403(r)(1)(B) and 403(r)(3) of this title or sections 403(r)(1)(B) and 403(r)(5)(D) of this title, is made in accordance with the requirements of section 403(r) of this title is not a drug solely because the label or the labeling contains such a claim. A food, dietary ingredient, or dietary supplement for which a truthful and not misleading statement is made in accordance with section 403(r)(6) of this title is not a drug under clause (C) solely because the label or the labeling contains such a statement.

The Food and Drug Administration further divides drugs into two categories, **synthetic drug** and **biologic**, depending on whether the compound is manufactured synthetically in a laboratory or derived from living sources such as humans, animals, and microorganisms. A synthetic drug is regulated by the FDA's Center for Drug Evaluation and Research (CDER) while a biologic is regulated by the FDA's Center for Biologics Evaluation and Research (CBER). In general, a synthetic drug is typically individual molecules that are synthesized in a pure state and then combined with chemical stabilizers and other ingredients to form a tablet or capsule. In contrast, biologics are often complex mixtures of ingredients that are not easily identified or characterized. In order for a drug or biologic to be approved for sale in the United States, a manufacturer must provide substantial evidence, usually the results of two well controlled clinical trials, that the substance is safe and effective for its intended use.

## VALUE AND USE

In the United States, drugs can be made available either with a specific prescription by a physician licensed to prescribe medicines (i.e., **prescription drug**), or sold directly to consumers as so-called **over-the-counter** (OTC) **drug**. For a variety of reasons, including the availability of insurance coverage for prescription drugs, OTC medications are more readily available and often less expensive than the prescription medications that require a physician visit and prescription.

The term **ethical drug** has been used to denote a product that was only advertised to physicians, a nomenclature that was derived from the 1847 code of ethics of the American Medical Association that precluded the advertising of physician services to the public. Since 1996, however, in the United States pharmaceutical companies have advertised directly to consumers, and this distinction has been lost. In general use, the term "ethical pharmaceutical" usually means a prescription drug.

The economic value of a drug is largely derived from the ability of the manufacturer to patent the product and restrict its manufacture and sale. In the United States, patents are generally applied for at the time of discovery and have a life of 20 years. The drug development process, from discovery to first sale, is a lengthy and costly process. As a result, the **effective patent life** is frequently significantly less than 20 years, and generally ranges between 8 and 12 years. Because of the rapid erosion of market share after patent expiration, some pharmaceutical companies have attempted to extend the life of their products by introducing a **line extension**. A line extension generally use the same active ingredient but offer additional consumer benefits through modifications in the delivery mechanism, such as an extended release formulation, rapid dissolving disks, and liquid suspension. In some cases, line extensions are created by combining one active ingredient with a second. In these cases, the patent protection on the combination is based on the longer-lived patent. Although manufacturers of generics are able to produce the original product, new patents protecting these line extensions enable the original company to retain a higher proportion of their market with the new products.

In 1984, the US government recognized that the drug application process was growing longer and longer and that this was reducing the incentive for firms to invest in research and development. To increase the incentives, Congress passed the Drug Price Competition and Patent Restoration Act. The act made it easier for a **generic drug** to be approved by reducing the burden of the application process and at the same time offering a patent extension of up to five years because of delays in the regulatory review process. A generic drug contains identical amounts of the same active drug ingredient as the brand name product and shows bioequivalence to the brand name product (*see term: Pharmacokinetics*), although it may differ in certain other characteristics (e.g., shape, flavor, or preservatives). Because of their complexity, biologics currently have no generic competitors. In the application process, a generic drug is shown to be "therapeutically equivalent," and hence it is assumed that they will have equivalent effects. In many states, pharmacists are empowered to substitute a generic drug for the prescribed brand name drug unless the physician indicates that the prescription must be "dispensed as written." As a result, after patent expiration, the sales of the brand name drug typically plummet. For example, in the first month after its patent ended in July 2001, the brand manufacturer lost over two-thirds of its market share of Prozac® to generic competitors.

Another way in which pharmaceutical companies compete with each other is through the introduction of branded "me-too" drugs. A **me-too drug** is a product that is in the same class as the original product (such as a statin or an ACE inhibitor). It generally has a similar molecular structure and purported mechanism of action as the original product and may offer some modest improvements in efficacy, safety, or convenience. Since good targets for potential therapeutic interventions become widely known, there is often a race among various manufacturers to bring the first drug in a new therapeutic class to market. Thus, second and third product entrants within a given class of products are often referred to as me-too drugs.

In some cases, two or more manufacturers hold a patent or license for a given product. This product is considered a **multiple source drug**, and there is an increased level of competition for it.

## Issues

In the United States, the Food and Drug Administration determines whether a product will be a prescription drug or an OTC drug. Because of the potential for unknown safety issues, new medications are almost always available first as prescription only. After gaining sufficient clinical experience, a manufacturer may request that a medication be made available directly to consumers. In many cases, because prices are higher for prescription drugs, manufacturers will delay requesting OTC status until the patent has expired or is about to expire. Recently, however, an insurance company requested that Claritin®, an allergy drug, be classified an OTC drug against the wishes of its manufacturer, in part because as an OTC drug it would no longer have to be covered by the company. The FDA eventually granted OTC drug status to the product.

There are also significant issues of public policy related to the question of patent life. On the one hand, patents create artificial monopolies and increase the cost of the medication to payers (insurance companies, governments, and consumers). On the other hand, these same rents create the incentives for pharmaceutical companies to invest millions of dollars in the development of such products. Thus, determining the appropriate balance between the short- and long-term benefits of patent policy plays an important and controversial role in the industry.

The creation of line extensions is also a topic of considerable debate. Critics of the pharmaceutical industry claim that these "new" products offer no additional benefits to patients but are merely an attempt by the industry to extend patents and continue to collect the monopoly rents. Defenders of the industry argue that these extensions must offer real benefits to patients and consumers, or they would simply not buy the newer products and would instead continue to use the cheaper, older, and now generic products. The issue is compounded by the effects of insurance (making patients and physicians less price sensitive) and the asymmetric information (patients relying on physicians' advice) that, some argue, distorts the ability of consumers to make knowledgeable choices about their pharmaceutical care. Adding to the complexity is the fact that many of the branded products are supported by significant sales and marketing efforts by the manufacturers, but once the patent expires these efforts cease. To the extent that these activities influence physician prescribing behavior, it is argued, physicians are biased toward prescribing the branded products even when equivalent products are available in generic form.

The creation of me-too drugs is also open to contention. Some critics of the industry suggest that these offer little therapeutic advantage over the existing products and therefore are a waste of precious research and development resources. They further argue that these products are used by the industry to perpetuate patent protection and generate profits. Alternatively, substantial evidence supports the position that me-too drugs offer clinical benefits to at least some patients because of subtle differences in formulation, dosing, and tolerability profiles; increase the level of competition in the industry; and result in increased patient access to beneficial treatments. Advocates further argue that it is very difficult to determine early on which specific product will ultimately meet patients' needs best, and therefore it is essential that there be research conducted on competing molecules; ending research with the first agent in a class, they say, would result in significant losses to patients.

BIBLIOGRAPHY

Abbott TA. *The Pharmaceutical Industry in Health Economics: Fundamentals and Flows of Funds.* Getzen TE, ed. New York: John Wiley and Sons, Inc; 1997.

Brown J. Quick Uptake: Generic competitors have devoured Prozac sales faster than Eli Lilly marketers had anticipated. *Med Ad News* 20; December 26, 2001: 26.

Generic Pharmaceutical Association. http://www.gphaonline.org. Accessed March 31, 2003.

Temin P. *Taking Your Medicine: Drug Regulation in the United States.* Cambridge, Mass: Harvard University Press; 1980.

The Code of Federal Regulations. http://www.gpo.gov/nara/cfr/index.html. Accessed September 24, 2003.

US Food and Drug Administration. Center for Biologics Evaluation and Research. http://www.fda.gov/cber. Accessed March 31, 2003.

Woodcock J. "Moving Forward: CDER." http://www.fda.gov/cder/present/Roundtable. Accessed April 2, 2003.

# Drug Efficacy
## Drug Effectiveness

BRIEF DEFINITION

**Drug efficacy** is a clinical outcome derived from patients' use of a pharmaceutical product in controlled settings, typically randomized control Phase I–III trials. Pharmaceutical regulatory agencies such as the Food and Drug Administration (FDA) rely upon these data to approve new drug products.

EXPLANATION

Before human testing can begin, preclinical development activities of drugs are required. The data collected for preclinical activities are the chemical name, structural formula, drug synthesis process, preparation methods, quality and purity data, dosage form identified, stability data, and toxicology studies including teratogenicity, carcinogenicity, and mutagenicity data performed on several animal species. When the preclinical development is complete, the sponsor applies to regulatory agencies for approval to begin human clinical trials. The pre-marketing clinical trials involve three phases, Phases I, II, and III. Phase I trials gather data to determine the safety profile and safe dosage range through pharmacokinetic and pharmacodynamic studies in up to 100 normal healthy volunteers. Phase II trials determine the optimum dose and evaluate efficacy and adverse event profiles through controlled studies in up to 500 patients. Phase III trials are larger, double-blinded, multi-center studies of up to 3000 patients to verify efficacy, safety, and long-term drug use, usually compared with a placebo in controlled studies. Once a regulatory agency approves a drug, it moves into Phase IV or postmarketing studies or surveillance where long-term safety and efficacy are evaluated through adverse event reporting and clinical trials. Safety and efficacy data are gathered in all types of controlled trials.

VALUE AND USE

A medical treatment needs to be safe and efficacious for human use. The approval process is designed to protect the public from dangerous and/or useless products. Safety and efficacy data provide highly scrutinized information for the health care provider to use in making decisions about treatment of patients, development of medical treatment guidelines, and evidence-based medicine.

ISSUES

There are three major drug efficacy issues. Do drug efficacy studies in a controlled environment represent the "real" environment? Do the drug efficacy studies detect drug adverse events adequately? Are drug efficacy studies needed for all substances used for medicinal use (i.e., herbal products).

With regard to drug efficacy studies representing the "real" word, the terms drug efficacy and **drug effectiveness** have been used interchangeably in the literature. Efficacy can answer, "Can it work under ideal conditions?" and effectiveness answers, "Does it work under real-world circumstances?" Usually efficacy studies are Phase II and III, in a tightly controlled clinical trial environment, whereas effectiveness studies are conducted during Phase IV, postmarketing studies or surveillance, in the real world environment.

With regard to drug efficacy studies detecting adverse events, in the United States, the FDA is under constant pressure to review Investigational New Drug Applications and New Drug Applications in an expeditious manner without compromising safety. This has advantages and disadvantages. As new drugs are approved and marketed, it is important for all health care providers to monitor for adverse events and report serious and unexpected events to the FDA's MedWatch program.

With regard to medicinal use of herbal products, in the United States, herbal products are regulated as dietary supplements. Manufacturers of herbal products that do not make a treatment claim for their product are not required to meet the FDA regulations of safety and efficacy. The FDA, however, does maintain a list of products that fall under the Generally Recognized as Safe (GRAS) category. This designation is based on the use as a food additive, not as a medicinal or therapeutic treatment. In Germany, the Federal Department of Health's Commission E reviews safety and efficacy of herbal products with monographs that describe the herbal's mechanism of action, medical uses, contraindications, adverse effects, drug interactions, administration, and dosage.

BIBLIOGRAPHY

CBER. www.fda.gov/cber/index.html. Accessed March 31, 2003.

CDER. www.fda.gov/cder/. Accessed March 31, 2003.

Dunsworth T. *Drug Regulatory Process. Pharmacotherapy Self-Assessment Program.* 2nd ed. Module 5. Kansas City, Mo: American College of Clinical Pharmacy; 1995.

Dunsworth T. *Drug and Practice Regulatory Issues. Pharmacotherapy Self-Assessment Program.* 3rd ed. Module 5. Kansas City, Mo: American College of Clinical Pharmacy; 1999.

FDA. www.fda.gov. Accessed March 31, 2003.

FDC Reports. www.FDCReports.com. Accessed March 31, 2003.

Kessler DA. The regulation of investigational drugs. *N Engl J Med* 1989;320:281–288.

MedWatch. www.fda.gov/medwatch/index.html. Accessed March 31, 2003.

# Drug Formulary

Drug Formulary System
Closed Formulary
Open-Preferred Formulary
Tiered Copayment
Open-Passive Formulary
Formulary Management

## BRIEF DEFINITION

A **drug formulary** is a continually updated list of medications that is preferred for use by a health system and will be dispensed through participating pharmacies to covered persons. The formulary is the product of the **drug formulary system**.

A drug formulary system is an ongoing process whereby a health care organization, through its physicians, pharmacists, and other health care professionals, establishes policies on the use of drug products and therapies, and identifies drug products and therapies that are the most medically appropriate and cost-effective to best serve the health interests of a given patient population.

## EXPLANATION

Health management organizations have used the formulary process since the 1970s. The formulary is typically the product of the organization's pharmacy and therapeutics committee review and evaluation process that seeks to guide physician prescribing through the inclusion of only selected products from the various drug classes. Drugs are usually chosen for formulary inclusion based upon an evaluation of published literature around the efficacy, safety, and tolerability of a drug compared with others (if applicable) within the same class. A pricing contract is then negotiated with the product manufacturer and factored into the decision. A formulary is typically classified as closed (or partially closed), open-preferred or open-passive. **Closed formulary** indicates that one or more classes of drugs are closed to only certain products. Only drugs included on the formulary in a closed class are covered by the drug benefit. **Open-preferred formulary** indicates an incentive-based system to encourage the use of preferred agents within the class. These incentives include lower copayments for the patient, academic detailing, and requests (usually in the form of a letter) to the physician to reconsider the choice of nonformulary drugs. Under this style of formulary, a **tiered copayment** approach is often employed. Under the tiered copayment system, the patient pays less for generic and progressively more for brand name and nonformulary drugs. A tiered formulary typically contains three to five tiers. An **open-passive formulary** indicates that few incentives are provided to encourage or change prescribing nonformulary drugs.

Formulary system decisions are based on scientific and economic considerations that achieve appropriate, safe, and cost-effective drug therapy. A formulary often contains information about available formulations and dosing but does not usually contain recommendations about the therapeutic use of the drugs.

## VALUE AND USE

When structured appropriately, the formulary can be a powerful tool in directing physicians to prescribe the most efficacious and cost-effective drugs to patients. The **formulary management** process is dynamic, with the formulary under constant review and revision as new products come onto the market and new data surface on existing drugs. A well designed and well-managed pharmacy and therapeutics committee can serve as an excellent source of expertise and guidance for the prescribing physician.

Moreover, several organizations have begun building outcomes criteria into the product review and evaluation process. These criteria can include: effectiveness (versus efficacy), quality of life, patient satisfaction, total cost of care (versus simply acquisition cost of the product), and workplace productivity.

## ISSUES

Many physicians see the formulary process as restrictive and cost-driven. In addition, because most physicians participate in multiple health plan provider networks, they must deal with the differing formulary of each of the entities. This can often lead to confusion, errors, and inefficiencies within the physician's practice that can undermine the physician's willingness to follow the formulary. It is only with the highest degree of standards and communications that these obstacles can be overcome.

## BIBLIOGRAPHY

Academy of Managed Care Pharmacy. *A Format for the Submission of Clinical and Economic Evaluation Data in Support of Formulary Consideration by Managed Health Care Systems in the United States.* Alexandria, Va: Academy of Managed Care Pharmacy; 2000.

The Coalition Working Group: Cahill JA, Fry R, Cranston JW, Zellmer WA, et al. *Principles of a Sound Drug Formulary System.* Formulary Management-Endorsed Document. Bethesda, Md: ASHP; 2000.

Goldberg RB. Managing the pharmacy benefit: the formulary system. *J Manag Care Pharm.* 1997;3:565–573.

Regence Washington Health Pharmacy Services. *Guidelines for the Submission of Clinical and Economic Data Supporting Formulary Consideration.* Seattle, Wash: Regence Washington Health; 1997.

# Drug Interaction

## BRIEF DEFINITION

A desirable or undesirable therapeutic consequence occurring when drugs are used in combination is a **drug interaction**. Drugs include pharmaceuticals, homeopathic drugs, nutritional food supplements, herbal products, chemicals, and diagnostic agents. Drugs can also interact with food or other substances.

## EXPLANATION

Pharmacologic interactions occur when the actions of one drug are altered by another drug or substance. Pharmacokinetic interactions occur when absorption, distribution, metabolism, or elimination of a drug is altered by another drug or substance. Mechanisms of drug interactions include but are not limited to the following:

1. Route of administration. Properties of drugs or chemicals given together, intravenously, may cause physical incompatibilities resulting in adverse events. Example: Calcium and phosphate products added to intravenous solutions are concentration-dependent, causing precipitation, with reports of death.

2. Drug metabolites. Metabolites of a drug may interact with another drug or its metabolites. Example: It is thought that erythromycin metabolite inhibits the metabolism of theophylline since increased theophylline levels are seen up to five days rather than in two to three days after starting erythromycin.

3. GI absorption and transport. Some drugs may bind with or inhibit the gastrointestinal absorption of another drug. Example: Antacids bind with tetracycline or ciprofloxacin resulting in decreased bioavailability of the antibiotic. Another important site for absorption and metabolism is the drug transport system mediated by P-glycoprotein (P-gp). This transport protein is found in the intestinal epithelium, renal tubule, liver, and blood brain barrier. Some drugs are enhanced while others are inhibited by the transport protein, changing the absorption and potential drug interactions of many drugs. Example: The current understanding for increased digoxin blood levels with quinidine is that quinidine inhibits P-gp, causing increased absorption and decreased renal clearance of digoxin.

4. Plasma-protein-binding interactions. One drug displaces another from the plasma-protein-binding sites, resulting in an increased level of free drug with increased pharmacologic effects. Example: Salicylates displace warfarin from plasma-protein-binding sites, causing an increased international normalized ration (INR) and effects, possibly including bleeding complications.

5. Metabolism. The most important organ for drug metabolism is the liver. However, drug metabolism also occurs in the gut, lung, skin, kidney, blood, and placenta. The cytochrome P-450 pathway is the leading enzyme pathway affected by many drugs. A drug may be classified as an inducer, inhibitor, or substrate. A substrate is a drug that is metabolized by a specific enzyme in the cytochrome P-450 pathway, which is affected by a second drug or metabolite, an inhibitor or inducer. The effects of drug–drug interactions can be predicted by knowing the enzyme metabolism pathway of the drug.
   - Enzyme-induction interaction. Certain drugs cause the liver to increase production of enzymes, resulting in rapid metabolism of the drug and lower blood levels and effects. Example: Cigarette smoking decreases theophylline levels. Rifampicin decreases drug levels of calcium channel blockers, cyclosporine, protease inhibitors, etc.
   - Enzyme-inhibition interaction. Certain drugs decrease the effects of enzymes that metabolize drugs. Therefore, less drug metabolized results in increased drug levels, possibly toxic levels. Example: Drugs that increase toxicity of cyclosporine are clarithromycin, diltiazem, fluconazole, grapefruit juice, etc.

6. Renal-excretion interaction. Drugs may compete for glomerular filtration, active tubular secretion, or passive tubular reabsorption, resulting in excessive blood levels of one or both drugs. Example: Probenecid de-

creases clearance of beta-lactams and causes increased levels and toxicity of methotrexate, rifampin, sulfonamide, sulfonylureas and zidovudine, etc.

7. Pharmacodynamic interactions. These occur when the pharmacologic properties of two drugs cause additive, synergistic, or antagonistic effects. Example: A narcotic analgesic and a benzodiazepine medication increase drowsiness, an additive effect. Carbidopa inhibits the metabolism of levodopa in the peripheral system, resulting in increased levels of levodopa crossing the blood brain barrier, a synyergistic effect. A hypertensive patient with controlled blood pressure receives a nonsteroidal antiinflammatory agent, which can cause fluid retention resulting in increased blood pressure, an antagonist effect.

## VALUE AND USE

The primary focus is the prevention or avoidance of morbidity and mortality caused by an interaction between two chemical entities.

## ISSUES

There are two major challenges for the health care professional: 1) keeping current with drug interaction information and 2) non-drug/drug interactions. Staying up-to-date with the literature on drug–drug interactions is a challenge. New information is constantly discovered. Drug–drug interaction-detecting software programs are available from various vendors. The validity of the software to detect clinically significant drug–drug interaction should be evaluated before implementation. Hazelet et al (2001) found the performance of programs tested to be suboptimal.

Although considered safe by the general population, many herbal products interact with pharmacological products. Example: St. John's Wort interacts with and decreases the effectiveness of protease inhibitor drugs. Also St. John's Wort may decrease the International Normalized Ratio (INR) for patients receiving warfarin.

## BIBLIOGRAPHY

Hansten PD, Horn JR. *Hansten and Horn's Drug Interaction Analysis and Management.* St. Louis, Mo: Facts and Comparisons Publishing Group; 2001.

Hazlet TK, Lee TA, Hansten PD, Horn JR. Performance of Community Pharmacy Drug Interaction Software. *J Am Pharm Assoc.* 2001;41:200–204.

Hunter J, Hirst BH. Intestinal secretion of drugs. The role of P-glycoprotein and related drug efflux systems in limiting oral drug absorption. *Adv Drug Deliv.* 1997;25:129–157.

Tatro DS, ed. *Drug Interaction Facts.* St. Louis, Mo: A Wolter Kluwer Company; 2001.

Slaughter RL, DJ Edwards. Recent advances: the cytochrome P450 enzymes. *Ann Pharmacother.* 1995;29:619–624.

# Drug Marketing
Opinion Leaders
Brand

## BRIEF DEFINITION
**Drug marketing** is the process of raising awareness and use of a pharmaceutical product.

## EXPLANATION
As with the adoption of any new technology, the adoption and use of new pharmaceuticals display a life cycle. There are early adopters who are advocates of the new medication and there are the late adopters—the health care providers who only use a medication well after it has become the standard of care. In between are the large majority of adopters or users. The goal of pharmaceutical marketing is to shift this curve to the left—that is, to accelerate the appropriate adoption and use of a new prescription pharmaceutical. Successful marketing efforts result in benefit both to the manufacturer—significant increases in sales and profits—and to society—many more appropriate patients achieve the benefits offered by the new medication.

The marketing practices of manufacturers are highly regulated. In addition, the market for prescription pharmaceuticals is characterized by imperfections including regulatory agency imperfections, asymmetries of information, and global sunk costs. These combine to reduce price sensitivity on the demand side, to enhance market power on the supply side, and to create demand curves that do not reflect societal benefits. Despite these important differences from other industries and markets, the pharmaceutical industry relies on many of the same principles applied in other markets to enhance the use of its products. Marketing and promotion are critical to raising awareness and use of any new product. Especially in the health care sector, information is "costly" and therefore many stakeholders—particularly physicians—are "rationally unaware" of a wide range of information. Physicians have high search costs for information about new therapies, since the data is often complex and their time is limited. Pharmaceutical promotion creates awareness of a new therapy, stimulates interest, explains attributes (benefits, side-effects), differentiates and positions the product, informs health care professionals, and sustains awareness. Promotion also includes education about the target disease and the range of treatments in addition to information about the marketed product.

Drug marketing strategies include development of a "brand" for a new product, characterization of the key medical specialties and **opinion leaders**, identification and prioritization of specific targets for market penetration based upon the profile of the new drug in comparison to existing therapies, and determining what is the best mix of promotional investments. The venues of promotion for prescription drugs largely consist of professional journal advertising, detailing by manufacturer sales representatives to physicians in their offices (including provision of samples), professional symposia and seminars, and more recently, direct-to-consumer advertising in various media, such as print, television, and others. Another component of marketing strategy is setting the price of the drug (*see term:* Drug Pricing).

Opinion leaders play an important role during the launch of a new product. They are usually nationally or internationally recognized experts affiliated with research or academic institutions. They usually are early adopters of new therapies and have the platform to influence the behavior of other practitioners.

For more than a century, the importance of branding in the pharmaceutical industry has been recognized; for example, Thomas Beecham named his new laxative "Beechams Pills." A **brand** is a name, term, sign, symbol, design, or combination of these that is intended to identify the goods or services of one seller or group of sellers and to differentiate them from those of competitors. Brands convey attributes, benefits, values, culture, personality, and characteristics of the user. A well-crafted brand imbues a product with brand equity— loyalty among its users. The importance of branding perhaps is most readily observed with the conversion of a growing number of drugs from prescription to over-the-counter status, in which direct-to-consumer (DTC) advertising has long been permitted. However, the building of brands was inherent in pharmaceuticals promotion prior to the advent of DTC advertising for prescription drugs in the United States. It is worth noting that the onset of DTC advertising for prescription drugs has largely resulted in a change in the mix of marketing investments rather than increases in total promotion budgets as popularly believed (Rosenthal et al 2002).

ISSUES

Direct-to-consumer advertising has become a lightning rod for public concerns over the rising costs of pharmaceuticals. Critics contend that manufacturers could lower drug prices if they reduced the costs associated with DTC advertising. This reflects a general ambivalence by the public toward pharmaceutical marketing: does it solely drive greater profits or does it also provide an important educational service to society? In addition, the pharmaceutical industry has come under fire for some of its promotional practices, including the provision of meals and gifts to physicians. The American Medical Association proposed a set of guidelines regarding the value of such gifts that has recently been embraced by the pharmaceutical industry. Perhaps of even greater concern is that some manufacturers are under investigation for potentially illegal activities to enhance the sales of specific products or to promote their use outside of approved indications. These developments have complicated public policy discussions about the appropriate role of pharmaceutical promotion, and have fueled calls for greater regulation of the pharmaceutical industry.

BIBLIOGRAPHY

Blackett T, Robins R, eds. *Brand Medicine: The Role of Branding in the Pharmaceutical Industry.* New York: Palgrave; 2001.

Dubois R. *Pharmaceutical Promotion: Don't Throw the Baby with the Bathwater Health Affairs.* Web Exclusive; February 2003. www.healthaffairs.org/webexclusives/dubois_web_excel_ 022603.htm. Accessed March 3, 2003.

Kotler P. *Marketing Management: The Millennium Edition.* Upper Saddle River, NJ: Prentice Hall; 2000.

Petersen M. Whistle-blower says marketers broke the rules to push a drug. *New York Times,* December 20, 2002: Section C; page 1 (col. 5).

Rosenthal M, Berndt E, Donohue J, et al. Promotion of prescription drugs to consumers. *New Engl J Med.* 2002;346:498–505.

# Drug Pricing
Pricing Strategy
Catalog Price
Average Wholesale Price
Rebates
Reference-Based Pricing
Differential Pricing

## BRIEF DEFINITION

**Drug pricing** is a complex process that aims to maximize access to new pharmaceuticals and the return on investment of pharmaceutical manufacturers. The prices in the US marketplace are set through interactions among manufacturers, wholesalers, retailers, insurers, and pharmacy benefit managers (PBM's). Internationally, prices may be set by governmental agencies that negotiate directly with manufacturers following the approval of the drug for marketing through their established regulatory review procedures. The **pricing strategy** developed by a manufacturer must balance the need to fund ongoing research and development in order to discover tomorrow's breakthrough medicines versus the need to make today's drugs available to those who need them.

## EXPLANATION

In the United States, the processes by which prices are determined and the final price paid for drugs by various purchasers vary immensely. The chain of distribution for a drug begins with the pharmaceutical company (manufacturer) that distributes the drug by selling to drug wholesalers, the middlemen between the manufacturer and the pharmacies. Using a value-based pricing model, a pharmaceutical company establishes a **catalog price** by considering a number of factors including: the value of the new drug in terms of treating disease and improving the quality of life, the value versus other available treatment options, the need to fund ongoing research and development, the need to provide a return to shareholders, and the need to provide access to the drug.

Frequently wholesalers may pay somewhat less than the catalog price for various reasons including timely payment. Wholesalers usually sell the drugs on a cost-plus basis to pharmacies (independents, chains, supermarkets, mail pharmacies, etc). The average price that wholesalers are paid is known as the **average wholesale price** or AWP. AWP is widely recognized as a benchmark and is acquired through a survey of wholesalers. However, it is clearly not what is paid at the pharmacy. After obtaining drugs through the wholesalers, pharmacies charge a mark-up to patients. The evidence that AWP is not the true price paid is evidenced by the typical reimbursement formula structured as AWP ± X% + dispensing fee. Pharmaceutical companies used to suggest AWP mark-ups (i.e., AWP + 15–25%), although these were not always followed. Pharmacies, the segment that is the primary customer for pricing service's estimates of AWP, benefit financially when the AWP + mark-up is relatively higher. Third party vendors, such as large managed care organizations or pharmacy benefit management companies, can frequently negotiate lower prices based upon the large volume of drugs that they use over their distribution networks. In the United States, for example, on average, for every dollar that a consumer pays for a prescription drug at the pharmacy, 74 cents goes to the drug manufacturer, 3 cents to the wholesale distributor, and 23 cents to the pharmacy. Other factors contribute to the wide differences in pricing, such as different pricing strategies between single source and multiple source drugs and between generic and brand name drugs.

Complicating the issue is the practice of **rebates**. Generally, when a MCO or PBM (*see terms*: Managed Care Organization, Pharmacy Benefit Management Organization) is considering adding, deleting, preferring, or prior-authorizing drugs from the formulary (a list of preferred drugs) (*see term*: Drug Formulary), it will negotiate with individual drug manufacturers about providing incentives or discounts off the negotiated price (a rebate) based upon its ability to move market share.

Internationally, governments or governmental agencies frequently negotiate drug prices. Increasingly manufacturers are being asked to provide pharmacoeconomic data to justify the requested price (*see terms*: National Institute of Clinical Excellence [NICE], Pharmacoeconomics). In some cases, countries have adopted a **reference-based pricing** policy. This may mean that a manufacturer may not be allowed to charge any more than the price of the least expensive drug currently marketed within a drug class (e.g., ACE inhibitors). It could also mean that a manufacturer cannot charge more than the price of the least expensive drug in a therapeutic category (e.g., antihypertensives). Reference-based pricing was introduced in Germany in 1989, The Netherlands in 1991, and Sweden and Denmark in 1993. Reference-based pricing is a mechanism to slow the increase in costs incurred by the government by the availability and use of new pharmaceuticals. The value of such a system is of considerable debate currently.

Developing a pricing strategy for a new product is a complex exercise and must take numerous factors into account, including the innovative value of the new drug compared to existing therapies, in order to determine the prices to be charged to various purchasers. Rarely is the cost of a drug's ingredients a significant factor in the pricing of a drug. Historical research and development expenditures have been invoked by some people as a significant factor in pricing a drug. For every 5000 medications evaluated, on average only 5 of these are tested in clinical trials and just one is approved for patient use; only 3 out of 10 drugs recoup or exceed their research and development costs. Thus revenues from successful drugs must fund the development of tomorrow's breakthrough drugs and the associated large number of failures. However, other people suggest that other factors are more important in drug pricing.

In setting the catalog price, the manufacturer must make a judgment of the value of the new product relative to existing treatments. When a new drug represents a significant advance over existing therapies (i.e., more effective, better tolerated), the price is usually set above the price of prevailing therapies. When a new drug is viewed as being little or no different from the product of competitors, the product may be priced equivalent to other products in the market. When a drug is viewed as equal to or slightly inferior to current or anticipated offerings, it may be priced below prevailing levels in hopes of gaining market share.

The pharmaceutical industry generally embraces a policy of **differential pricing**. Drugs are priced differentially to different customers to enhance access and utilization. For example, drugs sold to developing countries are priced lower than drugs sold to European countries. Within the United States, rebates are given to purchasers who provide care to large populations of patients and have demonstrated that they can influence drug utilization through formulary management techniques.

## VALUE AND USE

Product pricing strategies are reached in a number of ways and may change over time, during the life cycle of the product, and as other business needs change. Each product pricing decision is unique but should take into consideration a number of different factors, including the company history and position in the market, revenue goals, internal resources and capabilities, product features, past actions of the competition, target patient characteristics, disease characteristics, market position needs, the public policy environment, economic and social value of the therapy, and current and anticipated insurance reimbursement.

## ISSUES

Since most if not all pricing decisions should be market based, the assessment of the above factors are performed in an effort to understand customer value. Generally stated, customer value can be defined as customer-perceived benefits minus customer perceived costs (e.g., risks and price). Pricing strategies that do not provide customers with perceived value will not succeed.

## BIBLIOGRAPHY

Anderson F, McMenamin P. *International Price Comparisons of Pharamaceuticals—A Review of Methodological Issues.* London and Washington, DC: Batelle Medical Technology and Price Centre (MEDTAP); 1992.

Burstall ML, Reuben BG, Reuben AJ. Pricing and reimbursement regulation in Europe: an update on the industry perspective. *Drug Inf J.* 1999;33:669–688.

Danzon, PM. Making sense of drug prices. *Regulation.* 2000;23: 56–63.

Kolassa EM. *Elements of Pharmaceutical Pricing.* New York: The Haworth Press, Inc; 1997.

Leszinski R, Marn MV. Setting value, not price. *McKinsey Q.* 1997;1:98–115.

# Drug Research and Development

Basic Research                     Phase II
Preclinical Research               Phase III
Clinical Research                  Phase IV
Phase I                            Postmarketing Product Surveillance

**Drug research and development** consists of four stages:

1) Basic Research, 2) Preclinical Research, 3) Clinical Research (Phases I, II, and III), and 4) Postmarketing Product Surveillance (Clinical Research Phase IV)

## Basic Research

### BRIEF DEFINITION

The study of medicinal chemistry, pharmacology, physiology, disease states, and new technology for use in developing pharmaceutical products are referred to as **basic research**.

### EXPLANATION

For the development of medications and therapies, it is imperative that the underlying etiology of disease states be understood: What are the symptoms, how does the body respond to the disease, how does the body respond to an intervention? Basic pharmaceutical research focuses on understanding diseases and the impact of any interventions to diseases. In today's competitive environment, many thousands of compounds are synthesized and evaluated with precise bioactivity screens to select the few that will be pursued.

### VALUE AND USE

Basic pharmaceutical research has been a major impetus for our current understanding of the human body and the development of modern medicine.

### ISSUES

It is possible for knowledge produced from basic research to be exploited. Gene therapy is a frontier that promises to provide cures for many diseases. However, it is possible that the discovery of gene therapies will also produce technologies that can be used to the detriment of patients. For example, health insurance companies could use gene information to profile and refuse coverage to patients with "high risk genes."

## Preclinical Research

### BRIEF DEFINITION

**Preclinical research** is the laboratory and animal research conducted prior to any clinical testing of a new chemical entity.

EXPLANATION

Before a new compound can be tested in humans, research is needed to show that using the new compound is probably not detrimental to the health of humans. Therefore, research is performed with a new compound in at least two animal species. This research focuses on the safety of the new chemical entity and on the determination of doses that can be given without detrimental effects. Data from sophisticated animal models are used to design how the initial human trials will be conducted.

VALUE AND USE

Human clinical research would not be possible without preclinical research. It would be unethical to test new drugs in humans without knowing the safety profile in other species.

ISSUES

It is difficult to extrapolate results found in animal studies to humans due to the many physiological differences between animals and humans. Concerns of animal rights activists must also be addressed with regard to drug testing in animals. Whenever possible, animal tests are being replaced by other technologies.

## Clinical Research

BRIEF DEFINITION

Human testing of pharmaceutical products to evaluate safety and efficacy is known as **clinical research.**

EXPLANATION

There are four phases of human clinical research:

1. **Phase I.** Testing in a small number of healthy volunteers (e.g., 20–80). This testing determines whether there are any unanticipated safety issues that were not discovered during preclinical testing. Maximum safe doses, metabolic pathways, routes of elimination, and some evidence of biologic effect may be explored.

2. **Phase II.**
   - IIA. These dose-ranging studies are conducted in a somewhat larger sample (e.g., 75–100) of the target populations to determine appropriate doses that both exhibit biological effects and are well tolerated.
   - IIB. These are proof of concept studies, also in relatively large samples (e.g., 100–300) of the target population, in which evidence of efficacy (usually based upon biomarkers) and tolerability and safety are sought. Based upon the results of these studies, the dosage regimens are selected for Phase III studies.

3. **Phase III.** These are the pivotal large-scale studies (e.g., up to several thousand patients) in the target populations that support regulatory

approval for marketing of a new drug or a new indication for an existing drug. Usually two randomized placebo-controlled clinical trials are required to support regulatory approval, although single very large studies may be acceptable. Phase III studies increasingly include clinical endpoints (e.g., stroke, myocardial infarction, death) in addition to biomarkers (e.g., LDL-cholesterol, blood pressure). They may also include data on other outcomes (e.g., quality of life, health care utilization).

4. **Phase IV.** Separate studies such as **postmarketing product surveillance** studies may be conducted following the marketing of a new drug to evaluate various additional indications, the risk for particular adverse effects, the potential for differences in the drug's efficacy/safety profile in special populations or disease states (e.g., elderly, renal or hepatic insufficiency patients). In addition, studies may be conducted on alternate doses, dosing intervals, formulations, and combinations with other treatments, as well as head-to-head comparisons with particular drugs used to treat the same indicated conditions. Phase IV clinical research is the fourth stage of the drug research and development process.

## Value and Use

Clinical trials form the final basis for a drug's marketing approval. They determine how a drug will be used in humans. In addition to efficacy data, clinical trials provide valuable information pertaining to adverse effects, warnings, and precautionary information that is used in the product labeling.

## Issues

Clinical trials are time consuming, usually a minimum of three to five years. For serious disease states patient groups often criticize this lengthy process. Although it is difficult to shorten the timeline, drugs are often made available prior to approval for the very ill under strict regulatory procedures. Clinical and ethical issues have been raised about the appropriate comparator in Phase III studies. While use of a placebo provides the strongest evidence of a drug effect, it may not answer the questions of practicing clinicians, such as when should one use a new drug rather than existing therapies? Additionally, the use of placebo may not be ethical in some studies, especially when a condition is life threatening and alternative therapies are available.

## Bibliography

Getz KA, De Bruin A. Breaking the development speed barrier: assessing successful practices of the fastest drug development companies. *Drug Info J.* 2000;34:725–736.

Lesko LJ, Rowland M, Peck CC, Blaschke TF. Optimizing the science of drug development: opportunities for better candidate selection and accelerated evaluation in humans. *Pharm Res.* 2000;17:1335–1344.

Spilker B. Creating standards for basic, medical and market research. *Drug News Perspect.* 1998;11:197–203.

Spilker B. Reducing pharmaceutical risk. *Drug News Perspect.* 1998;11:325–330.

# Drug Safety
Adverse Event
Serious Adverse Event
Adverse Drug Reaction
Tolerability
Pharmacovigilance

## BRIEF DEFINITION

**Drug safety** involves the assessment, management, and communication of the risks involved in the use of a pharmaceutical agent. In general, there are two phases of drug safety: preapproval and postapproval drug safety. Preapproval drug safety relies primarily on clinical trial data; postapproval drug safety utilizes information from voluntary spontaneous reports, postmarketing surveillance (e.g., registry), and population-based epidemiological data for purposes ranging from signal detection to risk quantification to causality evaluation.

## EXPLANATION

The risk associated with use of a pharmaceutical product is measured by adverse events or side effects. An **adverse event** (AE), opposite to drug therapeutic effect, is an undesired or unintended medical condition or sign temporally associated with the use of an approved or investigational pharmaceutical product, whether or not causally related to the product. An AE meets the definition of a **serious adverse event** (SAE) when an AE results in death, is life threatening, requires inpatient hospitalization or prolongation of existing hospitalization, results in persistent or significant disability/incapacity, or is a congenital anomaly/birth defect. **Adverse drug reaction** (ADR) is an undesired pharmacological effect that within a reasonable possibility is causally related to the use of a pharmaceutical agent. (This definition excludes accidental or deliberate excessive dosage or misadministration.) The causation may have a pharmacological plausibility or be of an idiosyncratic nature.

In the preapproval phase, **tolerability**, which represents the degree to which overt side effects of a pharmaceutical agent can be tolerated by study subjects, is assessed in clinical trials. Tolerability is partly reflected by the rate of discontinuation from the trial due to adverse events.

Despite the vigorous scientific standard for proving efficacy and safety in the preapproval phase, controlled clinical trials have inherent shortcomings and may have limited generalizability to the real world environment in which medical practice occurs. Clinical trials (that support initial registration) are conducted in a controlled setting with restrictive inclusion and exclusion criteria, seldom involve more than 2000 patients, and the study duration is limited to weeks, months, or at most, a limited number of years. Uncommon side effects or delayed adverse reactions of long-term administration may not be observed. Moreover, many of the patients who are most likely eventually to be exposed to the pharmaceutical agent often are not studied in this setting. This includes the elderly, pregnant women, children, and patients with multiple concurrent diseases who are taking several concomitant medications. Postmarketing surveillance, therefore, is crucial for providing additional safety information that cannot realistically be collected before approval of a drug. A key component of such surveillance is the voluntary reporting of spontaneous ADRs. The scientific field of collecting, analyzing, and interpreting the postmarketing spontaneous reports is termed **pharmacovigilance**. Pharmacovigilance is intended to generate, detect, and/or validate signals for potential side effects from marketed products based on the numerator data (i.e., ADR reports). At times, a product withdrawal decision by a regulatory agency could hinge on a few spontaneous reports demonstrating high causal correlation. More scientifically vigorous methods of hypothesis-testing of the causality of such events would involve the conduct of large-scale population-based pharmacoepidemiology studies (*see term:* Pharmacoepidemiology). Some researchers also include epidemiological studies of drug safety in the field of pharmacovigilance.

## Value and Use

Drug safety is one side of the risk-benefit analysis when determining whether to use pharmaceutical agents. Only when the benefit of using a pharmaceutical agent is judged to outweigh the risk, as evaluated by patient's medical care provider, is the use of the agent warranted.

## Issues

The data used for drug safety assessment, including clinical trials data, postmarketing spontaneous reports data, and population-based observational data, have their own strengths and weaknesses. The clinical trials data are of high accuracy but have limited generalizability to the real-life user population. Postmarketing spontaneous reports data are generated through a passive surveillance system that relies on voluntary reporting of adverse events from conscientious, astute health professionals and consumers. They therefore tend to be under-reported, difficult to quantify because of the lack of a denominator, and the reported AE cases may be a biased subset of all existing cases. Large computerized population-based databases would enable the quantification of causation between the pharmaceutical agent and AE by allowing the identification of an at-risk population and the selection of comparison groups. However, the accuracy of population-based data may not be as high as clinical trials data.

## Bibliography

*A Dictionary of Epidemiology.* 3rd ed. New York: Oxford University Press; 1995.

Edwards IR. Spontaneous ADR reporting and drug safety signal induction in perspective. *Pharmacol Toxicol.* 2000;86(suppl):S16–19.

Fletcher AP. Spontaneous adverse drug reaction reporting vs event monitoring: a comparison. *J R Soc Med.* 1991;84:341–344.

Mann R, Andrews E, eds. *Pharmacovigilance.* Chichester, UK: John Wiley & Sons; 2002.

Sills JM, Tanner LA, Milstien JB. Food and drug administration monitoring of adverse drug reactions. *Am J Hosp Pharm.* 1986;43:2764–2770.

Talbot JC, Nilsson BS. Pharmacovigilance in the pharmaceutical industry. *Br J Clin Pharmacol.* 1998;45:427–431.

# Drug Use Evaluation
Drug Use Review
Medication Use Evaluation
Prospective Drug Use Evaluation
Concurrent Drug Use Evaluation
Retrospective Drug Use Evaluation

## BRIEF DEFINITION
**Drug use evaluation** (DUE) is a criteria-based, ongoing, structured, organizationally authorized process designed to improve the appropriate, safe, and effective use of drugs.

## EXPLANATION
Drug use evaluation (DUE), **drug use review** (DUR), and **medication use evaluation** (MUE) are terms commonly used to describe the review of medication use in individual patients and large patient populations either by individual pharmacists or by formal processes established by health care delivery systems (hospitals, managed care organizations, etc). The terms drug use evaluation, drug use review, and medication use evaluation, and its predecessor term antibiotic utilization review (AUR), each emerged as products of initiatives, accrediting organizations, or legislation developed to address the growing concern about drug appropriateness, safety, and cost. The drug evaluation movement grew as the use complexity and cost of medications took more visible roles in clinical and political debates regarding health care quality and affordability.

Today, the terms DUE, DUR, and MUE are commonly interchanged. In practice, drug evaluations or reviews are commonly viewed as quality-assurance activities that focus on evaluating and improving medication-use processes with the goal of optimal patient outcomes and cost. In all cases, formal drug reviews or evaluations are criteria-driven. The criteria are developed and approved by a committee (i.e., health care providers). The methodology of the evaluation and outcome measures is clearly delineated. The results and outcomes are reported back to the committee. These data, with committee action and follow-up, would be part of the organization's quality improvement program for accreditation by various organizations. (e.g., in the United States, Joint Commission on Accreditation of Healthcare Organizations, National Committee for Quality Assurance).

Drug evaluations or reviews are classified in three categories:

**Prospective Drug Use Evaluation**: evaluation of a patient's drug therapy before a medication is dispensed

**Concurrent Drug Use Evaluation:** ongoing monitoring of drug therapy during the course of treatment or at the point of dispensing

**Retrospective Drug Use Evaluation:** review of drug therapy after the patient(s) has (have) received the medication

## VALUE AND USE

DUE/MUE helps to identify actual and potential medication-related problems, resolve actual medication-related problems, and prevent potential problems that could interfere with achieving optimum outcomes for patients.

DUE programs play a key role in helping managed health care systems understand, interpret, and improve the prescribing, administration, and use of medications with the goals of improved patient outcomes and more efficient use of scarce health care resources. Pharmacists play a key role in this process because of their expertise in the area of pharmaceutical care. DUE affords pharmacists the opportunity to identify trends in prescribing within groups of patients such as those with asthma, diabetes, or high blood pressure. As a result, pharmacists can, in collaboration with physicians and other members of the health care team, initiate action to improve drug therapy for both individual patients and covered populations.

## ISSUES

By their very nature drug use evaluation studies are local. They are administrative surveys carried out to monitor and correct local practices. As such, they may have limited research value beyond their geographic and temporal borders. Additionally, the pharmacist conducting the DUE may not have adequate or complete data to evaluate the patient's medication therapy. For example, a community (retail) pharmacist may not have access to the patient's laboratory data to evaluate renal or hepatic function for the appropriate dose. Electronic systems can significantly improve access to patient data.

Nevertheless, these reviews can provide useful data for studies that attempt to examine the factors that determine inappropriate drug use.

## BIBLIOGRAPHY

Cahill JA, Cranston, JW, Zellmer WA, Principles of a Sound Drug Formulary System Coalition Working Group, et al. Formulary management. *Amer Soc Hosp Pharm.* 2000:139.

Joint Commission on Accreditation of Healthcare Organizations. *Accreditation Manual for Hospitals.* Chicago: Joint Commission on Accreditation of Healthcare Organization; 1992.

Navarro R, Wertheimer AI. *Managing the Pharmacy Benefit.* Wayne, NJ: Emron Publishing; 1996.

Ninno MA, Ninno SD. Quality improvement and the medication use process. In: Malone PM, Masdell KW, Kiar KL, Stanovich JE, et al, eds. *Drug Information. A Guide for Pharmacists.* Columbus, OH: McGraw-Hill; 1996:445–479.

# Effect Modification
## Effect Modifier

### BRIEF DEFINITION
**Effect modification** refers to a situation in which the association between the exposure and the disease under study varies by levels of a factor (*see term:* Epidemiology). This factor is called an **effect modifier.**

### EXPLANATION
If we divide the study population into two distinct categories or strata, the stratum-specific effect measures may or may not be equal. If they are equal, we say that the effect measure is homogeneous, constant, or uniform across strata. If they are not equal, we say that the measure is heterogeneous or modified across strata—that is, the effect of exposure on disease varies over this factor. For example, there is an increased risk for thromboembolism among women who use oral contraceptives (OC) as compared to women who do not use these pills. With respect to smoking, the relative risks for thromboembolism among women using OC is not the same. Those OC-users who smoke have a statistically increased risk as compared to the nonsmoking OC-users. We have an effect modification with respect to the association between use of oral contraceptives and thromboembolism where smoking is an effect modifier.

### VALUE AND USE
From a public health perspective, information on effect modification can be used to identify special risk groups—for example, users of oral contraceptives who smoke, which could be targeted for preventive actions. Information on effect modification can also be used to learn more about and to test hypotheses of biological relationships.

### ISSUES
The term "effect modification" is closely related to the concept of interaction, which has been somewhat controversial in the epidemiological literature. An assessment regarding the presence or absence of effect modification depends on how one defines the state of no-effect modification. Statistical analysis of effect modification or term interactions must be considered (*see term:* Uncertainty). Multiplicative models and additive models have been used to assess different biological models. The concept of effect modification should not be confused with the concept of confounding (*see term:* Epidemiology).

BIBLIOGRAPHY

Hennekens CH, Buring JE. *Epidemiology in Medicine.* Boston: Little, Brown and Company; 1987.

Kleinbaum DG, Kupper LL, Morgenstern H. *Epidemiologic Research. Principles and Quantitative Methods.* New York: Van Nostrand Reinhold Company; 1982.

Rothman KJ, Greenland S. *Modern Epidemiology.* Philadelphia: Lippincott-Raven Publishers; 1998.

# Epidemiology

Natural History
Risk Factor
Sociodemographic Factor
Descriptive Epidemiology
Cross-Sectional Study
Analytic Epidemiology
Cohort Study

Case-Control Study
Risk Ratio
Retrospective Study
Odds Ratio
Population Attributable Risk
Bias
Confounding

BRIEF DEFINITION

**Epidemiology** is the branch of public health that works to understand the distribution, causes, and effects of disease in communities. Epidemiologists study the factors and relationships that determine the presence, numbers, trends, and distribution of diseases in communities and in specific populations.

EXPLANATION

Epidemiology translates from the Greek as the science of that which exists in the population. Epidemiology originated in the nineteenth century as the study of infectious disease distribution and the analysis of probable causes of epidemics; epidemiology was and is very important in developing preventive measures in public health. The causal factor per se (bacteria, virus, prions, chemicals, etc) need not necessarily be known in order to use epidemiological findings to identify population groups at risk and to perform interventions or give health advice to avoid further disease development.

VALUE AND USE

The basic question asked in the pioneering studies was: What factors do those with disease have in common that individuals who remain healthy do not have?" This is still the basic issue in epidemiological studies even though epidemiology has expanded into the study of virtually every type of disease or outcome at a population or group level; epidemiology now also refers to the specific methodology and reasoning used in population studies. Epidemiological methods are also used to study the distribution, causes, and effects of use of medicines in the population (pharmacoepidemiology) (*see term:* Pharmacoepidemiology) as well as the effects of environmental exposures (e.g., pollution).

Epidemiology can be used to study the **natural history** of diseases—that is, the development and outcome of untreated disease. Thus, epidemiology today is concerned not only with disease as the only outcome; the methodology also can be used in the study of a variety of outcomes and exposures in health care research.

A **risk factor** (*see terms:* Risk, Risk Adjustment) is a factor whose presence is associated with an increased likelihood that disease or another outcome studied will develop at a later time. Disease and injury in populations vary relative to many factors such as age, race, sex, occupation, geography, living conditions, income, residence, exposure, and genetic predisposition; this type of factor is called a **sociodemographic factor**.

There are two basic types of epidemiological study design: descriptive and analytical. A **descriptive epidemiology** study aims to describe the incidence (*see term:* Incidence), prevalence (*see term:* Prevalence), mortality (incidence of death) (*see term:* Health Status) or fatality (incidence of death in diseased individuals) morbidity rates for diseases or injuries in a population. Descriptive studies include what is called a **cross-sectional study**, which is a study performed at one point in time and aims to study the correlation between risk factors and outcomes in a defined population. Ideally, data on exposure and outcome should be known at an individual level; studies that utilize aggregated statistics (vital statistics, drug sales data, etc), however, may be prone to ecological fallacy—that is, spurious correlations.

**Analytic epidemiology** studies take the time perspective into consideration; they are designed to verify that the suspected exposure did in fact occur before the outbreak of disease. The main types of analytical studies are the **cohort study** and the **case-control study**.

In the cohort study, a prospective study (*see term:* Clinical Trial) as shown in the figure, individuals who are exposed and those who are nonexposed to the suspected causal agent in a defined population are followed forward from the time of exposure, and incidences of the outcome are determined in the two groups. The ratio of incidence in exposed divided by the ratio of incidence in nonexposed gives the relative risk or **risk ratio** (RR) (*see term:* Risk) for developing the outcome.

In the case-control study, a **retrospective study** as shown in the figure, individuals with the disease or outcome of interest are identified as one study group and individuals from the same population without the outcome are used as the control group, with the intent being to mirror the rate of the outcome

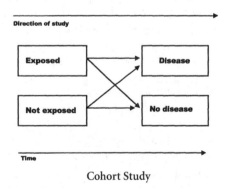

Cohort Study

in the population (*see term:* Retrospective Analysis). The two groups are then retrospectively studied to identify any possible causal exposures. The relative risk of the outcome cannot be determined directly, since the population

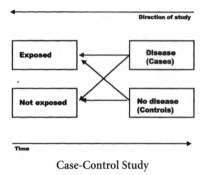

Case-Control Study

incidences are not known (*see term:* Risk). The relative risk is therefore approximated through the **odds ratio** (OR), that is, the odds for being exposed among the diseased divided by the odds for being exposed among the controls. It has been shown that for outcomes with a relatively low prevalence—which is most outcomes—the odds ratio is a satisfactory estimate of the relative risk.

In an epidemiological study, it is also possible to estimate the attributable risk (AR) and the **population attributable risk** (PAR) (*see term:* Risk). The AR gives information on the excess risk of disease among the exposed compared with those nonexposed and is calculated as the incidence among exposed minus the incidence among unexposed. The PAR is defined as the excess rate of disease in the population that is attributable to exposure under study. It is calculated as the incidence of disease in the total population minus the incidence in the unexposed.

ISSUES

Since epidemiological studies are performed in nonrandomized, noncontrolled environments, there are several important methodological considerations in epidemiological studies. Epidemiological studies can be, and often are, subject to **bias,** that is, systematic errors that result in incorrect estimates of the association between exposure and outcome studied. There are a great number of potential

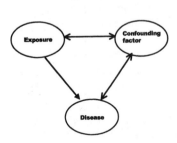

The Relationship between
Exposure, Confounding Factor,
and Disease

sources of bias in a study, the most common being selection bias (bias in the way study subjects are selected) and information or observation bias (systematic differences in the way information on exposure and/or outcome is obtained in the groups studied) (*see terms:* Clinical Trial – Study Bias, Sample Selection Model). Bias should be controlled as far as possible in the design of the study, and the possible effects of bias should always be discussed in the evaluation of study results.

Another important alternative explanation for the association found in an epidemiological study is **confounding**. Confounding refers to the effect of the exposure under study being mixed with the effect of a third factor. The third factor must be a risk factor for the disease as well as associated with the exposure, as shown in the figure. Common confounding factors include age and sex. Confounding can be controlled in the study design through randomization, restriction (inclusion criteria), or matching. Confounding can also be evaluated and controlled in the analysis through stratified analysis or multivariate methods.

BIBLIOGRAPHY

Barker G, Rose DJP, Coggon D, ed. *Epidemiology for the Uninitiated.* London: BMJ Books; 2003.

Beaglehole R, Bonita R, Kjellstrom T. *Basic Epidemiology.* Geneva: World Health Organization; 1993.

Hennekens CH, Buring JE. *Epidemiology in Medicine.* Boston: Little, Brown and Co; 1987.

Rothman K, Greenland S, eds. *Modern Epidemiology.* 2nd ed. Philadelphia: Lippincott-Raven; 1998.

# European Medicines Evaluation Agency (EMEA)

Centralized Procedure
Mutual Recognition Procedure
Committee for Proprietary Medicinal Products

The **European Medicines Evaluation Agency** (EMEA) was founded January 1, 1995. EMEA coordinates centralized drug registrations for the European Union market as a whole. This **centralized procedure** exists along with the **mutual recognition procedure** and the national registration procedures for drugs. For scientific tasks, EMEA has two key committees: the **Committee for Proprietary Medicinal Products** (CPMP) and the Committee for Veterinary Medicinal Products (CVMP). Only the former will be considered here.

Based in London, the EMEA coordinates the scientific assessment of new biological and chemical entities, which follows the centralized procedure for European Union registration. This scientific assessment comprises three major aspects: quality, preclinical and clinical safety, and effectiveness. The several hundreds of employees of the EMEA are not involved in the scientific assessment procedures as reviewing experts, but they coordinate the centralized registration procedure. In addition to the centralized procedure, the EMEA has several other tasks, including postmarketing surveillance (PMS), provision of product information, development of guidelines, and publication of opinion papers. The EMEA's tasks in PMS involve judgment and dissemination of information on adverse drug effects. The scientific assessment for proprietary medical products and all other scientific assessment during the postmarketing phase are under the responsibility of the scientific committee—the CPMP.

The CPMP consists of two delegates per member state. Delegates are assigned by the national authorities for a period of three years. The CPMP's drug evaluation must be finalized within 210 days from the moment that the EMEA has verified receipt of the files from the pharmaceutical company involved. The CPMP issues an opinion to approve or reject the drug application. This opinion is transposed into a legally binding decision by the European Commission (EC), involving a standing committee with member state representation. Normally the EC decision will comply with the CPMP opinion. The final authorization is valid throughout the whole European Union.

The centralized procedure is obligatory for new biopharmaceuticals and optional for other products of an innovative nature such as new chemically active substances. Next to the centralized procedure, a second option for drug registration exists in the mutual recognition procedure for products intended for more than one member state. This procedure is executed by the National Drug Authorities with the help of a voluntary group, the Mutual Recognition Facilitation Group (MRFG), which meets at the EMEA. The mutual recognition procedure involves the request of a pharmaceutical industry to register a drug in one or more member states on the basis of the registration already achieved in another member state (known as a reference member state or RMS). During the first four years of the procedure, it has been applied almost 500 times. The United Kingdom was most often selected by pharmaceutical companies to act as the RMS.

The national procedures can still be used for products intended for one market only; as soon as a pharmaceutical company wishes to register the same product in another member state, though, the mutual recognition procedure must be used.

BIBLIOGRAPHY

EMEA. www.emea.eu.int. Accessed March 31, 2003.

# EuroQoL
## EQ-5D

BRIEF DEFINITION

EuroQoL, also referred to as EQ-5D, is a generic instrument for measuring health-related quality of life, designed to be self-completed by the respondent. It has been in the public domain since 1990. The EuroQol group developed this instrument to complement other health-related quality of life measures. EuroQol has four components: description of the respondent's health by means of the classification, rating of his/her health by means of a "thermometer," valuation of a set of health states, and background information about the respondent.

EXPLANATION

The EuroQoL group was established in 1987. The original members came from various research teams in Europe. The group was multilingual and multidisciplinary. In 1994, the EuroQoL group was reconstituted into an association with members from not only Europe but also other continents.

The EuroQol is a questionnaire with several sections. On page 2 (self-identifier), the respondents are asked to describe their own health state on the following five dimensions: mobility, self-care, usual activities, pain/discomfort, and anxiety/depression. Each dimension provides three levels from which the respondents can choose. On page 3 (visual analogue scale method), respondents are asked to indicate their own current health state on a "thermometer" calibrated from zero ("worst imaginable health state") to 100 ("best imaginable health state"). Pages 2 and 3 are the only parts of the instrument that need to be used if the researchers are interested only in measuring the health-related quality of life of the patient. If the researchers are also interested in establishing valuations, they need to ask the respondents to value 13 standard health states, again on 0–100 thermometers, on pages 5 and 6. After this, on page 7, the respondents are instructed to go back to pages 5 and 6 to draw a line to mark off the position of the state "dead" compared to the other states. Pages 8 and 9 contain questions eliciting background information from patients, including age, sex, education, disease experience, smoking status, and so on.

## Value and Use

Based on the description above, the self-classifying section (page 2) of EuroQol can be defined by a five-digit number. For example, the state 22223 indicates some problems with mobility, self-care, usual activities, and pain/discomfort, and extreme problems with anxiety/depression. Since there are three choices for each dimension, there are potentially $3^5 = 243$ health states according to this classification. The data of self-reported problems can be used as a profile of health status. The information from this section of EuroQol can also be used to derive a single summary index. In addition, researchers have used the ratings from the visual analog scale as a measure of outcome. In past studies, the EuroQol self-identifier and the visual analog scale have been used in a variety of ways: comparing patients' health status at different times; assessing the seriousness of illness at different times; providing effectiveness evidence for approval of drugs or processes; providing relevant resource allocation information at different levels; and establishing local and national population health status. EuroQol has been used in quite a number of clinical areas.

## Issues

Several issues are worth noting with respect to EuroQol. The first is that such a simple instrument as EuroQol is not likely to be comprehensive and sensitive in measuring health status, although the developers incorporate a visual analog scale to cover the whole health state spectrum from worst to best.

The second issue arises with valuation of standard health states. It involves several aspects, the first of which is the duration of health states. The EuroQol designers opted to present the health states to patients as lasting one year. However, the prognosis for a state, the probabilities of death, and the difference in time preference of different respondents could all influence the valuation of health states. The second aspect of the valuation issue is the number of health states to value. Although empirical work has placed emphasis on valuation of the standard health states, the EuroQol group has continued to explore the possibilities of valuing other health states. The third aspect of the valuation issue of EuroQol is the approaches of valuation. A visual analog scale has been used for simplicity but there is evidence that a visual analog scale does not provide cardinal values or utilities. Thus, the EuroQol group felt it important to explore other possible valuation approaches.

The third issue is the methodological requirements of EuroQol. First is the instrument's practicality: using pages 2 and 3 of EuroQol is a convenient way to describe and rate respondents' current health status, but the valuation of standard health states has not been considered easy. Besides practicality, the reliability, validity, and response bias aspects of EuroQol also need to be considered.

The fourth issue emerges when "dead" is valued by respondents, who clearly have difficulty in the valuation of this "state."

BIBLIOGRAPHY

Brooks R. EuroQol: the current state of play. *Health Policy.* 1996;37:53–72.

Kind P, Dolan P, Gudex C, Williams A. Variations in population health status: results from a United Kingdom national questionnaire survey. *BMJ.* 1998;316:736–741.

Rabin R, de Charoo F. EQ-5D: a measure of health status from the EuroQol group. *Ann Med.* 2001;33:337–343.

# Evidence-Based Medicine

Cochrane Collaboration
Centre for Reviews and Dissemination
Evidence-Based Practice Centers

## BRIEF DEFINITION

**Evidence-based medicine** has been defined as an approach to health care practice in which the clinician is aware of the evidence in support of his or her clinical practice and of the strength of that evidence and is then able to apply that knowledge in clinical practice. Evidence-based medicine, therefore, consists of clinical expertise and patient preferences combined with critical appraisal of clinical research, with the goal of providing optimal individual patient care. Optimal care thus takes into account patient outcomes and the relative efficiencies among competing alternatives, as demonstrated in the medical literature. This approach to patient care demands that the clinician's expertise and the appraisal of the clinical evidence base be current and up to date.

## EXPLANATION

Historically, clinical care has been provided based on clinical expertise and some notional review of the clinical literature. Today, there is an ever increasing burden on clinicians to keep up with relevant literature and advances in their respective fields as both the body of medical literature and clinical advances continue to expand and accelerate. Additionally, health care delivery systems are under pressure to provide state-of-the-art medical interventions, but in the most efficient manner. To help balance these twin burdens, evidence-based medicine (EBM) is being increasingly pursued as a rational approach to patient care.

EBM requires that clinicians have access to critical, unbiased reviews of currently available evidence. One especially visible example of early efforts to review literature in a systematic way is the **Cochrane Collaboration**. This effort was begun in response to the suggestion by a British epidemiologist, Archie Cochrane, that critical, systematic and up-to-date reviews of all relevant randomized controlled trials in health care were needed to fully realize the potential of medical research for patient care. Cochrane Centres across the world engage in the production of Cochrane reviews according to a specific methodology. Many other research bodies conduct rigorous systematic reviews, among which, for example, are the **Centre for Reviews and Dissemination** (CRD) at the University of York in the United Kingdom and **Evidence-Based Practice Centers** (EPCs) funded by the Agency for Health care Research and Quality (AHRQ) in the United States.

VALUE AND USE

The need for and value of EBM is increasingly being recognized. It is appearing more frequently in medical school curricula and postgraduate workshops, and medical journals are now devoted to EBM. The academic courses include teaching critical appraisal of the literature so that clinicians become savvier regarding individual published studies and reviews. Also, since the late 1980s, there has been a large increase in the number of written clinical practice guidelines produced that use the principles of systematic reviews together with expert clinical opinion to help inform patient-level decision making. Like EBM as used in clinical practice, clinical practice guidelines take into account the knowledge gained through experience of clinicians and typically reflect local or regional practice. Systematic reviews focus less on experiential evidence and rely instead on evaluation of clinical trials and aggregation of their results to make conclusions concerning the evidence. The goal of EBM is to enable physicians to obtain and take unbiased sources of information into the patient encounter and use them in the clinical decision-making process. It is a basic tenet of EBM that patient specific characteristics and preferences be explicitly considered.

ISSUES

Although the goal of EBM reviews and guidelines is to be timely, current, and unbiased, EBM in actuality is also sometimes criticized for not having those characteristics. Sometimes, reviews and guidelines are criticized for not being timely and not reflecting current knowledge. As well, controversy exists as to what clinical literature deserves to be included in the reviews and depended upon for the guidelines. For example, some argue that only randomized controlled trials (RCTs) should be included, while others maintain that such trials suffer from external generalizability and other issues and can be supplemented and complemented by a variety of outcomes studies, especially in the absence of trial data. Similarly, some maintain that only indexed literature has the quality to be included, while others maintain that the "gray" (nonindexed) literature may be included if it meets predetermined criteria for inclusion. Of course, that increases the intensity and scope of EBM reviews, and their concomitant expense. Overall, however, it is critical that such reviews be of the highest quality. If they are not, the field risks being perceived as simply another cover for decision makers merely trying to reduce or contain costs with inadequate evidence. This concern highlights the importance of an unbiased treatment of the evidence base. Impartial reviewers and adherence to standard procedures can help mitigate these concerns. It should also be noted that the most expensive treatment may in fact be the most efficient in improving patient outcomes.

## BIBLIOGRAPHY

Guyatt GH, Haynes BR, Jaeschke RZ, et al. For the Evidence-Based Medicine Working Group. Users' guides to the medical literature: XXV. Evidence-based medicine: principles for applying the users' guides to patient care. *JAMA.* 2000;284:1290–1296.

Sackett DL, Rosenberg WMC, Gray JAM, et al. Evidence based medicine: what it is and what it isn't. *BMJ.* 1996;312:71–72.

Sackett DL, Straus SE, Richardson WS, et al; Meyer HS, ed. Evidence-Based Medicine: How to Practice and Teach. *General Practice.* 1995;45(8398):506.

# Food and Drug Administration (FDA)

### BRIEF DEFINITION

The US **Food and Drug Administration** (FDA) is the regulatory authority that has responsibility for the approval of new drugs, biologics, and devices through the Center for Drug Evaluation and Research (CDER), the Center for Biologics Evaluation and Research (CBER), and the Center for Devices and Radiological Health (CDRH).

### EXPLANATION

The US Congress passed the Food and Drugs Act in 1906, which made it illegal to distribute misbranded or adulterated foods, drinks, and drugs across state lines. In 1938, Congress passed the Federal Food, Drug, and Cosmetic Act, which required companies to prove the safety of new drugs before putting them on the market. The new act also added the regulation of cosmetics and therapeutic devices. Since the early 1960s, the Food and Drug Administration has required that drugs used in the United States be both safe and effective. In 1997, Congress passed the Food and Drug Administration Modernization Act, which reauthorized the Prescription Drug User Fee Act of 1992 and mandated the most wide-ranging reforms in agency practices since 1938. Provisions included measures to accelerate review of devices, regulate advertising of unapproved uses of approved drugs and devices, and regulate health claims for foods.

### VALUE AND USE

FDA reviews the results of laboratory, animal, and human clinical testing done by companies to determine if the product they want to put on the market is safe and effective. Premarket review is conducted for new human drugs and biologics, complex medical devices, food and color additives, infant formulas, and animal drugs. Once products are on the market, FDA keeps track of how they are manufactured and responds to reports of adverse experiences or newly identified risks. If monitoring turns up a problem that needs to be corrected, FDA can ask the manufacturer to recall the product, or it can withdraw approval (of a drug, for example), require labeling changes, or send warnings to physicians or other health practitioners. The FDA also monitors the marketing practices of pharmaceutical companies to ensure that promotion is accurate, balanced, and does not make claims inconsistent with the approved labeling.

ISSUES

The FDA policies aim to preserve the high efficacy standard required for marketing drugs in the United States. However, once a drug is approved for marketing, a physician can use it in any fashion that he or she deems appropriate. The FDA must balance the risks and benefits associated with approval of new products for medical use. Since complete information about the full spectrum of risks and benefits is not usually known at the time of approval, risk management has received greater attention recently, and the FDA is asking manufacturers to develop risk management strategies to accompany the launch of new products.

BIBLIOGRAPHY

Federal Food, Drug, and Cosmetic Act of 1938 (21 USC §301-95).

# Gene Therapy
Somatic Gene Therapy
Germline Gene Therapy

## BRIEF DEFINITION

**Gene therapy** is a novel approach to treat, cure, or ultimately prevent disease by changing the expression of a person's genes. Gene therapy is in its infancy, and current gene therapy is primarily experimental, with most human clinical trials only in the research stages. Gene therapy can be targeted to somatic (body) or germ (egg and sperm) cells. In **somatic gene therapy** the recipient's genome is changed, but the change is not passed along to the next generation. In **germline gene therapy**, the parents' egg and sperm cells are changed with the goal of passing on the changes to their offspring. Germline gene therapy is not being actively investigated, at least in larger animals and humans, although a lot of discussion is being conducted about its value and desirability.

## EXPLANATION

Cells may be modified ex vivo for subsequent administration to humans, or may be altered in vivo by gene therapy given directly to the subject. When the genetic manipulation is performed ex vivo on cells, which are then administered to the patients, this is a form of somatic cell therapy. Somatic cell therapy is the administration to humans of autologous, allogeneic, or xenogenic living cells that have been manipulated or processed ex vivo. The process involves the ex vivo propagation, expansion, selection or pharmacologic treatment of cells, or other alteration of their biological characteristics, such as genetic manipulation.

Genetic manipulation may be intended to have a therapeutic or prophylactic effect, or it may provide a way of marking cells for later identification (diagnostic purpose).

Recombinant DNA materials used to transfer genetic material such as genetically modified viral vectors are considered components of gene therapy. Other ways to apply gene therapy include liposome-encapsulated DNA, antisense techniques, naked DNA injection, DNA-mismatch repair, stem cell therapy and xenotransplantation of genetically modified animal cells. This list is not exhaustive, and still other ways are currently under investigation.

Distinction is also made between gene therapy focusing on germline and on nongermline cells. Within the area of germline cells, investigators prefer to use the word "genome modification" instead of gene therapy. The former may also include genome therapy, prevention, and genome enhancement, although it may be difficult to make clear distinctions among them. For instance, genetic intervention that avoids the birth of a child with cystic fibrosis would be regarded as gene therapy and/or prevention, whereas genetic intervention to increase the height of an otherwise normal future child would be genetic enhancement.

Different degrees of genome modification ranging from substituting a single nucleotide to changing a whole gene or chromosome are possible.

## VALUE AND USE

Gene therapy holds the promise of enabling the diagnosis and treatment of a variety of diseases for which there are currently no available effective therapies. It also potentially may lead to cures for common chronic diseases that require chronic or lifelong treatment. However, at the present time gene therapy is still experimental and therefore its benefits and risks remain to be shown.

The benefits of gene therapy may include disease prevention, reduction of disease severity, improved functioning, improved quality of life, and increased longevity. The harms may have a wide and very severe range not only for the patient, but also for future generations in case of germ cell modification with a bad outcome such as premature death.

## ISSUES

Gene therapy is still in its infancy stage. It is expected that in the near future specific regulations for the different types of gene therapy will be considered: how, when, and under which condition the trials may occur. Gene therapy also raises a host of ethical issues. According to Brenner and Moen (1996) some of these include:

- What is normal and what is a disability of disorder, and who decides?
- Are disabilities diseases? Do they need to be cured or prevented?
- Does searching for a cure demean the lives of individuals presently affected by disabilities?
- Is somatic gene therapy more or less ethical than germline gene therapy?
- Preliminary attempts at gene therapy are exorbitantly expensive. Who will have access to these therapies? Who will pay for their use?

## BIBLIOGRAPHY

Brenner MK, Moen RC. *Gene therapy in cancer.* New York: Marcel Dekker, Inc; 1996.

Guidance for industry. Guidance for human somatic cell therapy and gene therapy. *Hum Gen Ther.* 2001;12:303–314.

Human Genome Project Information—Gene Therapy. http://www.ornl.gov/hgmis/medicine/genetherapy.html. Accessed March 31, 2003.

Regulatory issues. Health department of United Kingdom gene therapy advisory committee. *Hum Gen Ther.* 2001;12:711–720.

Resnik DB, Langer PJ. Human germline gene therapy reconsidered. *Hum Gen Ther.* 2001;12: 1449–1458.

# Health Care Intervention
Medical Technology
Health Technology
Preventive Intervention
Primary Preventive Intervention
Secondary Preventive Intervention
Tertiary Preventive Intervention
Diagnostic Intervention
Therapeutic Intervention

## BRIEF DEFINITION

According to the MeSH (Medical Subject Headings) definition, **health care intervention** is a generic term used to describe a program, policy, measure, or activity designed to have an impact on an illness or disease in an individual or a population.

## EXPLANATION

The entire spectrum of health care intervention activities aims at promoting and preserving health, maintaining and restoring good health to the extent technologically possible, and preventing the departures from health that impair the well-being and working ability of individuals and communities.

In a real sense, all diagnostic and therapeutic activity (interventions) has a preventive component in that it seeks to interdict deterioration of the patient's health or forestall spread of disease, both infectious and environmental, in the community. Thus, prevention is often inseparable from treatment and cure. Many factors influence individual and systematic health care interventions. These include the historical and cultural context, which determines the values of society; available facts about perceived human need, which is defined and influenced by social values; and scientific and technical capability to intervene effectively.

Following the definition of technology as "the systematic application of scientific or other organized knowledge to practical tasks," the US Office of Technology Assessment has defined **medical technology** as "devices, and medical and surgical procedures used in medical care and the organizational and supportive systems within which such care is provided."

The term **health technology** is broader than medical technology in that it includes interventions encouraging consumer behaviors most likely to optimize health potential, both physical and psychosocial, through health information, preventive programs, and access to medical care technology. Health technology is classified not only by its nature—that is, drugs, devices, or procedures—but also by medical or health purpose. Health purpose can be diagnosis, prevention, therapy, rehabilitation, administration, or support (e.g., hospital beds or food services).

**Preventive intervention** is said to have three components: primary, secondary, and tertiary. **Primary preventive intervention** is directed toward preventing the occurrence of disease or injury, for example by immunization against infectious diseases and by the use of safety equipment to protect workers in hazardous occupations. Examples of other primary preventive interventions include health education, improved nutrition, and appropriate care for women during pregnancy.

**Secondary preventive intervention** means early detection and intervention, preferably before the condition is clinically apparent, and has the aim of reversing, halting, or at least retarding the progress of a condition. It is epitomized in screening programs in which people with early, often preclinical, manifestations of disease are identified and offered a regimen to prevent its progression. In other words, secondary preventive interventions are measures seeking to arrest or retard disease through early detection and appropriate treatment or to reduce the occurrence of relapses and the establishment of chronicity, through, for example, rehabilitative measures, corrective surgery, and the provision of prostheses. Examples include neonatal detection of congenitally dislocated hips and phenylketonuria.

**Tertiary preventive intervention** is undertaken to minimize the effects of disease and disability by surveillance and maintenance aimed at preventing complications and premature deterioration. Examples include the use of splints and remedial exercises to prevent contractures and deformities associated with rheumatoid arthritis, and care of pressure points and bladder function in paraplegia.

In epidemiological terms, primary prevention reduces the incidence of disease, secondary prevention reduces the prevalence, while tertiary prevention alleviates the effects.

**Diagnostic intervention** is defined as an organized service for the purpose of providing diagnosis to promote and maintain health and to identify therapeutic interventions necessary to treat the established illness. Each disease category encompasses the diagnostic interventions relevant for detecting its specific symptoms, manifestations, and severity. Diagnostic interventions might be noninvasive (rather, less invasive), moderately invasive, and heavily invasive. Urinary laboratory tests that do not involve catheterization are examples of less invasive diagnostic interventions. On the other hand, biopsies, although diagnostic, are considered as surgical, invasive interventions. Among the moderately invasive diagnostic interventions, one would list such procedures as densitometry, mammography, pneumoradiography, tomography, ultrasonography, and echocardiography.

**Therapeutic intervention** includes the following components: pharmacological intervention (efficacious agent of relevant dose, administration, and duration), therapeutic surgical intervention, and specialty care administered or provided by a health care professional. Therefore, therapeutic interventions are combinations of provider skills or abilities with drugs or devices or both. Examples of surgical therapeutic interventions include angioplasty, balloon dilation, balloon occlusion, central venous catheterization, and heart catheterization. Administration of a respiratory ventilator is an example of a specialty care administered by a trained health care professional.

## VALUE AND USE

Efficacy, safety, and efficiency are the basic starting points in evaluating the overall utility of most health care interventions. If an intervention is not safe, it should not be used, and if its efficacy is not known, statements about its value cannot be made. Information about the efficacy of existing and new health care interventions is also needed to determine cost-effectiveness and to guide public policies that develop, adopt, and use health care interventions. Such information could potentially be used to ensure that health care interventions demonstrated to have potential benefits with acceptable risks are made available rapidly, to constrain the diffusion and use of interventions which either lack efficacy or cause excessive harm, and to guide appropriate use of all interventions.

For example, labeling information along with the physician's skills and experience guide therapeutic interventions. Physicians use their own knowledge and the patient's reactions to make judgments regarding the applicability of a therapeutic intervention in each individual case, taking into account labeling data on clinical pharmacology (mechanism of action and pharmacokinetics), indications and uses, dosages for different types of patients, available forms of therapy, contraindications, precautions, side effects and adverse reactions, special considerations, patient and family education, and monitoring parameters. The developed information is meant for health professionals, and it explains the efficacy of a drug (pharmacological intervention) and alerts them to certain dangers and restrictions in its use. The US Food and Drug Administration's regulations on labeling ensure a high standard of safety and efficacy of marketed drugs.

## ISSUES

There is virtually no diagnostic or therapeutic intervention that is not potentially harmful to some degree. In the evaluation and treatment of every patient, the physician must continually balance these risks against the magnitude of the disease he or she is attempting to diagnose or treat. These accumulated risks have been referred to as the price we pay for modern management of disease. The bulk of information presently available concerns the acute toxic or other adverse side effects of diagnostic and therapeutic interventions. The long-term effects are largely unknown. The acute adverse effects of drugs do not represent the totality of the risk they present to the patient. Our "ignorance" in this area must be and has been acknowledged by the evolution of scientific methods evaluating health care interventions and their respective outcomes in more scientific ways.

Our definition of benefits and outcomes expands beyond measuring mortality and morbidity. Life expectancy, quality of life, and psychosocial and functional benefits have entered the domain of measurable outcomes. As a society comes to value these benefits more, we can anticipate more studies that attempt to measure them and that can be used in developing policies on specific health care interventions. Studies examining and comparing costs and cost-effectiveness of health care interventions are equally important.

BIBLIOGRAPHY
Kilbourne ED, Smilie WG. *Human Ecology and Public Health.* 4th ed. London: The MacMillan Company, Ltd; 1969.
Last JM. *Maxcy-Rosenau Public Health and Preventive Medicine.* New York: Appleton-Century-Crofts of Prentice-Hall, Inc; 1986.
US Office of Technology Assessment. *Medical Technology and the Costs of the Medicare Program.* Washington, DC: Office of Technology, Assessment; 1984.

# Health Care Payer
Single Party Payer
Third Party Payer

BRIEF DEFINITION
A **health care payer** is the party responsible for the financing and payment of health care for a population of eligible persons.

EXPLANATION
Understanding a health care system should include an examination of consumers (patients), health care providers, and the financing mechanism. The most prevalent models of health care payment include single and third party payment. In a **single party payer** system, a single agency or government pays for everyone's health care using tax revenue. **Third party payer** includes an organization, private or public, that pays for or insures at least some of the health care costs of its beneficiaries. An example of third party payers includes managed care organizations or systems (e.g., health maintenance organizations) that receive payment from individual patients, public agencies (such as Medicaid), or private entities (such as employers) seeking to secure health benefits for a population of persons that they represent. The third party will arrange a network of physicians and other providers that will provide health care services for the population of persons covered by the third party for a negotiated price (*see term:* Managed Care Organization). The figure below illustrates the relationship among the third party, the patient, and the provider.

At the broadest level the essential features of managed care are that: (1) the functions of health insurance and health care purchasing are integrated within the same organization and (2) health care is funded prospectively (i.e., so much

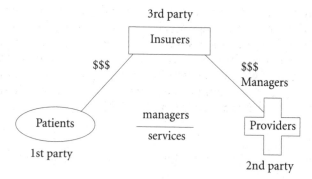

Example of a third party payment system: a managed care
scenario in the United States

per person or group to be covered) rather than retrospectively (i.e., fees for
treatments already purchased).

### VALUE AND USE

All countries face the issue of trying to balance the desire for economic efficiency with comprehensive, high-quality health services. An understanding of
who the principal "payers" are within a health care system helps us to gain an
appreciation of the possible sources of conflict that exist between the broadly
public and private organizations or agencies funding, and in some instances
providing, health care.

### ISSUES

Identifying the main payers of health care is an essential requirement to understanding how different countries are managing and responding to increasing
financial pressures. Challenges include the introduction of new and expensive
health care technologies (often for previously untreatable conditions) and
financing health care for an ever growing elderly population. Understanding
these challenges is critical to establishing the necessary research questions and
study design to describe the value of health care technologies.

### BIBLIOGRAPHY

OECD Health Data. 2000 Edition. The reform of health care systems: A review of seventeen OECD
    countries. In: OHE Compendium of Health Statistics. 12th ed. Paris: OECD; 2000.

## Health Care Payment System

### BRIEF DEFINITION

A **health care payment system** is the mechanism for reimbursing various providers of health care for the services that they provide in the delivery of health care.

## EXPLANATION

Providers might receive "payment" for the services they provide by one or more of the following methods:

- Fee-for-service (FFS), i.e., fee per case (per diem or flat rate)
- Capitation
- Salary
- Reimbursement (prospective or retrospective) or refund

A further framework for understanding provider "reward" systems is to consider the specific features of public and private health care provision in terms of (1) ownership of facilities and (2) employment and payment of general practitioners, as shown in the table.

**Public and Private Provision**

| Country | Ownership of Facilities | Employment and Payment of General Practitioners |
|---|---|---|
| Canada | Private not-for-profit | Mainly fee-for-service (FFS), some salaried |
| Germany | Mixture of public and private (for-profit and not-for-profit) | Mainly FFS outside hospital, salaried in hospitals |
| Netherlands | Private not-for-profit | Hospital: FFS<br>General practitioners: capitation and FFS |
| Sweden | Almost all public | Salaried public service |
| Switzerland | Mixture of public and private | General practitioners: mainly FFS<br>Hospital: salaried<br>A few Health Maintenance Organizations (HMOs) (most still insurance-owned group practices): doctors salaried. |
| UK | Mainly public, plus some private for-profit and not-for-profit | Hospital: salaried in the public sector<br>FFS in private practice<br>General practitioners are independent contractors (recently reorganized as preferred provider groups)<br>Mixture of salary, capitation, and FFS |
| USA | Mainly private (for-profit and not-for-profit) supplemented by public | Moving from mainly FFS to capitation and salaried |

Mounting financial pressures in recent years have created even more cost-conscious health care decision makers. The need for increased efficiency (i.e., value for money) and productivity balanced with quality improvement (partly as a result of the increasing consumerism in health care) reflects the reality of the scarcity of resources in all health care systems striving to deliver "evidence based" health care (i.e., taking account of both clinical and cost-effectiveness issues).

VALUE AND USE

A knowledge of the main methods for describing provider reward systems is a necessary prerequisite in understanding some of the important differences in country-specific health care systems.

Furthermore, any analysis of sources of health care finance and finance mechanisms has important implications for the design, conduct, and interpretation of economic evaluation studies of new treatments, technologies, drugs, etc. The perspective that is taken is also an important consideration (e.g., from the perspective of only the payer of health care or of society as a whole). The transferability of results is often problematic, and therefore such studies should always be made country-by-country.

ISSUES

A key issue relates to the relationship of financial incentives and distribution of monies (e.g., from state funds, insurance organizations, patients themselves) across all the players involved in providing health care and the relationship of these financial incentives to the access, quality, and cost of health care. For example, the influence of different financial incentives on practitioners' behavior in the traditional fee-for-service reimbursement system is well known. The incentive here is to do more because more services lead to more revenue.

BIBLIOGRAPHY

Chen GJ, Feldman SR. Economic aspect of health care systems. Advantage and disadvantage incentives in different systems. *Dermatol Clin.* 2000; 18:211–214.

Finkler SA. The distinction between costs and charges. *Ann Intern Med.* 1982:96:102–109.

*OECD Health Data. 2000 Edition. The reform of health care systems: A review of seventeen OECD countries.* In: *OHE Compendium of Health Statistics.* 12th ed. Paris: OECD; 2000.

# Health Care Provider

Primary Care Provider
Secondary Care Provider
Tertiary Care Providers
Allied Health Personnel

BRIEF DEFINITION

The term **health care provider** covers all health professionals, groups of health professionals, and health care organizations that provide services to patients in order to prevent or cure diseases, stop their progression, or ease disease-related symptoms.

EXPLANATION

A common classification divides general health services and consequently health care providers by the levels of care: primary, secondary, and tertiary care. According to this scheme, **primary care provider** covers basic health care for simple and common illnesses and injuries—in other words, routine health care needs. Primary care providers typically include generalist physicians such as family practitioners as well as internists, pediatricians, ophthalmologists, and even gynecologists.

Patients whose conditions require more specialized or skilled services may seek the care of a specialist—that is, a **secondary care provider**. Specialists are physicians specially trained in certain branches of medicine related to specific services or procedures (e.g., radiologists), certain age categories of patients (e.g., geriatricians), certain body systems (e.g., cardiologists or urologists), or certain types of disorders (e.g., allergists). Specialists usually limit their services to the area they have extensive knowledge of. Secondary care can be provided in an inpatient (hospitals) as well as in an outpatient setting. Under the last heading fall services provided in ambulatory care centers, outpatient departments of hospitals where the patient does not stay overnight, or physicians' practice offices.

A third level of care comprises **tertiary care providers**. These are "specialized specialists," providers who have extensive knowledge and skills in medical subspecialties. For instance hand surgeons, vascular surgeons, neurosurgeons, and pediatric endocrinologists are providers on the tertiary care level. In many countries these services are provided in specialized clinics or in university hospitals, since in most cases they require sophisticated equipment and support services.

At all three levels of care, **allied health personnel** also act as health care providers. These are health workers qualified by training and often by licensure to assist, facilitate, or complement the work of physicians. Their daily work sometimes also includes administrative services. Although the tasks of allied health personnel can show high degrees of specialization, their services generally do not require the high level of academic education that physicians have. Examples are surgical technicians, respiratory therapy technicians, nurses, and midwives.

## VALUE AND USE

The last century experienced a rapid increase of medical knowledge. Wide specialization patterns in the provision of medical services have largely been a function of these diagnostic and therapeutic advances. In this respect, the distinction between primary, secondary, and tertiary care providers gives one a classification system that allocates health care professionals or organizations according to their level of specialization to different provider groups. This classification system is helpful in international comparisons of health care systems and the availability of resources (e.g., the numbers of physicians, organizations, or hospital beds). Additionally, a classification of health care providers according to different specialization levels is helpful in the investigation and the comparisons of the cooperation patterns between health care providers in different countries (e.g., in examining how integrated or fragmented care is in a particular health care system).

Issues

The main issues related to the health care providers include the supply, access, and cost of care provided by health care providers. For example, many countries, in attempting to lower costs, may limit the access to secondary and tertiary providers. In this strategy, primary care providers act as "gatekeepers" to the health care system. Different methods are employed to achieve this goal. While in some countries reimbursed access to secondary or tertiary providers is only possible with a referral from a primary physician (e.g., in the British National Health System), other models offer insured patients lower insurance premiums if they refrain from self-referrals and agree to see specialists only on their primary physician's advice (e.g., a reform perspective for the German "Krankenkassen" or common practice in managed care organizations).

Bibliography

Godber E, Robinson R, Steiner A. Economic evaluation and the shifting balance towards primary care: definitions, evidence and methodological issues. *Health Econ.* 1997;6:275–294.

Jegers M, Kesteloot K, De Graeve D, Gilles W. A typology for provider payment in health care. *Health Policy.* 2002;60:255–273.

Mills A, Drummond M. Value for money in the health care sector: the contribution of primary health care. *Health Policy Plan.* 1987;2:107–128.

# Health Economics

Brief Definition

**Health economics** is a discipline that analyses the economic aspects of health and health care and that usually focuses on the costs (inputs) and the consequences (outcomes) of health care interventions using methods and theories from economics and medicine.

Explanation

The overall objective of health economics is the study of the economic aspects of all activities designed to improve or maintain health. This includes methods of financing health care; manufacturing health care products; training health care workers; identifying health care needs; and evaluating, distributing, and using health care products and interventions. Health economics employs principles of ethics, quality, utility, efficiency, and equity.

The discipline has two perspectives: positive and normative. From the positive perspective, health economics is based on rational behavioral models, production function, supply, demand and market adjusted to the characteristics of health care services. It takes into account consumer behavior in the health care sector and attempts to determine consumers' reactions to specific changes. From the normative perspective, health economics studies the efficiency, economic planning, and economic outcomes of health care policy in order to establish priorities and select strategies.

Pharmacoeconomics (*see term:* Pharmacoeconomics) is a discipline that employs health economics, pharmacoepidemiology, and health outcomes research methods to determine the costs and outcomes of health interventions, primarily pharmaceuticals. The aim is to provide information that can lead to a more efficient use of health care resources, bearing in mind the above-mentioned principles.

## Value and Use

Health economics is becoming increasingly important as health care expenditures rise due to an increase in chronic diseases relative to imminently life-threatening diseases, the aging of the population, and the availability of costlier and more complex health care interventions. For this reason, the authorities, the private health care insurance companies, and the health care industry itself are all interested in developing and applying a discipline that will supply data that contribute to a more rational and efficient use of limited health care resources.

## Issues

Health economics uses economic, pharmacoepidemiological, and health outcomes research methodologies and tools. For this reason, it should be considered as not just a branch of economics, but as a multidisciplinary specialty interrelated to economics and health care sciences.

## Bibliography

Gold MR, Siegel JE, Russell LB, et al. *Cost-Effectiveness in Health and Medicine.* New York: Oxford University Press; 1996.

Johanneson M. *Theory and Methods of Economic Evaluation of Health Care.* Dordrecht, The Netherlands: Kluwer Academic Publishers; 1996.

Kielhorn A, Graf JM. *The Health Economics Handbook.* Tattenhal, UK: Adis International; 2000.

# Health Insurance

**Premium**
**Benefit Design**
**Certificate of Coverage**
**Third Party Administrator**
**Deductible**
**Copayment**

## Brief Definition

**Health insurance** combines individual risks across a population and serves to reduce the uncertainty in the amount that an individual spends on medical care each time period (e.g., one year).

## Explanation

For an individual, medical illnesses may appear to strike randomly. When it does occur, an illness may impose a large burden and lead to high costs of treatment. Health insurance is a program for pooling the risks associated with the uncertainties of medical illnesses and the resulting expenditures for medical care. In exchange for a certain amount of money, called the **premium**, the insurer will cover a set amount of medical expenses should health services be required. The premium must be paid periodically to keep the policy in force or active. Because people tend to be risk-averse, they are willing to pay the premium to avoid the chance of having to pay a large amount when illness occurs.

The description of services available for patients for the premium paid is generally referred to as the **benefit design** while the legal disclaimer of the services available is described in the **certificate of coverage**.

## VALUE AND USE

According to the law of large numbers, the average from many individual events, each of which may be largely unpredictable, can be forecast reasonably well. Hence, by operating on a large-scale basis, an insurer can achieve a lower level of risk than is faced by an individual. Since people generally do not like risk, the purchase of insurance can improve well-being and maintain living standards by protecting the individual against the possibility of having to pay the total costs of receiving medical care. The risk-spreading nature of insurance is the source of its social value. The health insurance program may be administered by the government, a private insurance company, or a **third party administrator** (TPA). A TPA is an individual or company that contracts with employers that self-insure the health of their employees. The TPA develops and coordinates the insurance program, processes and pays claims, and may locate stop-loss insurance for the employer group.

## ISSUES

The design of an efficient health insurance program must contend with issues beyond the pooling of risks. For instance, moral hazard refers to changes in individuals' behavior that occur once they are insured because they are no longer liable for the full cost of those behaviors. An example is the overconsumption of medical care when an insured person makes unnecessary visits to a health care provider. The insurance policy may contain provisions that put some of the responsibility back onto the insured individual in order to curtail these behaviors. A **deductible** is the amount of medical care expenditures incurred by the insured individual (and/or any covered dependents) that are borne by the enrollee before the insurer begins making payments. Deductible requirements vary by plan and policy, and are in force over the course of a set period. A **copayment** is a form of cost sharing whereby the insured person pays a specified amount of the medical care. The copayment can be a fixed amount (e.g., $10 per drug prescription) or a percentage of the bill (e.g., 20% of a hospital bill). The covered person is usually responsible for payment at the time the service is rendered.

BIBLIOGRAPHY

Cutler DM, Zeckhauser RJ. The anatomy of health insurance. In: Culyer AJ, Newhouse JP, eds. *Handbook of Health Economics*. Amsterdam: Elsevier; 2000.

Folland S, Goodman AC, Stano M. *The Economics of Health and Health Care*. 2nd ed. Upper Saddle River, NJ: Prentice Hall; 1997.

Santerre RE, Neun SP. *Health Economics: Theories, Insights, and Industry Studies*. Chicago: Irwin; 1996.

# Health Insurance Programs, Government – United States

Medicare
Medicaid
Medicaid Prudent Pharmaceutical Purchasing Act
Centers for Medicare and Medicaid Services (CMS)

## BRIEF DEFINITION

**Government supported health insurance programs in the United States** are called **Medicare** and **Medicaid** (for other than military personnel or military veterans). Medicare is a federal government program to provide health care coverage to individuals aged 65 or greater, disabled workers, and individuals with end-stage renal disease. Medicaid is a program jointly funded by the federal and state governments to pay for medical care for certain individuals and families with reduced financial capabilities. The **Medicaid Prudent Pharmaceutical Purchasing Act** (MPPPA) is a federal law enacted as part of the United States' Omnibus Budget Reconciliation Act of 1990 (42 USC 1396r-8. Payment for Covered Outpatient Drug), that mandates that pharmaceutical companies must offer the Medicaid programs prices equivalent to the best discounted prices of any institutional drug purchaser.

## EXPLANATION

Created in 1965 as an amendment to the 1935 Social Security Act, Medicare is the primary health insurance plan that covers the elderly and the disabled in the United States. The plan comes under the auspices of the **Centers for Medicare and Medicaid Services (CMS)**, formerly the Health Care Financing Administration). Currently, it covers 39 million Americans.

Medicare comprises two distinct components. Part A (hospital insurance) can be seen as the basic foundation of the plan. This is financed through employee and employer tax contributions, trust fund interest, and beneficiary cost sharing (premiums, deductibles, copayments). Medicare is the primary source of insurance for those aged 65 or greater, covering the majority of beneficiary costs (55.1% of the total costs covered by Medicare). Patients automatically become eligible for Part A upon turning age 65. Part B (medical insurance) is an optional additional coverage that patients can receive. The majority of patients choose to receive Part B because it covers physician and outpatient services. By also covering skilled nursing facilities, hospice care, and home health care, this

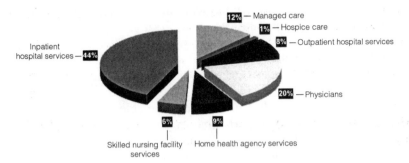

**Services Covered by Medicare - 1997**

Managed care 12%
Hospice care 1%
Outpatient hospital services 8%
Physicians 20%
Home health agency services 9%
Skilled nursing facility services 6%
Inpatient hospital services 44%

component is especially appealing to the elderly. Unlike Part A, a regular premium is paid per month for Part B. The overall coverage provided through Parts A and B is significant, as illustrated in the figure.

The Medicaid program was instituted in 1965 by Title XIX of the Social Security Act as a jointly funded, cooperative venture between the federal and state governments. Its purpose is to assist the states in providing adequate medical care to residents who cannot afford it. The federal government sets broad national guidelines within which each state's program must operate. Each state then establishes its own criteria for eligibility; determines what services will be provided; sets the reimbursement rates; and administers its program.

To receive federal matching funds, a state program must provide basic services. These include hospital, physician, laboratory, and X-ray services; nursing facility and home health care services for adults; family planning, pediatric, and family nurse practitioner services; rural health clinic services; screening, diagnosis, and treatment services for people younger than age 21; and other services according to rules that are subject to change. States may also receive federal funding for various other optional services and devices, such as eyeglasses, prosthetic devices, and dental services.

Some Medicare beneficiaries may also receive help from the Medicaid program for services such as nursing facility care beyond the 100-day limit covered by Medicare, prescription drugs, eyeglasses, and hearing aids. Services covered by Medicare are reimbursed by Medicare before payments are made by Medicaid.

In accordance with the MPPPA, pharmaceutical companies are asked to charge Medicaid programs, via a rebate mechanism, no more than the lowest price charged to hospitals or other organizations serving the underprivileged. For example, these rebates can be either 15.1% of average wholesale price (AWP; a benchmark set by the drug companies by which insurers base payment) of a given product or the difference between AWP and the "best price" for which a manufacturer sells a product, whichever is greater.

## VALUE AND USE

Aside from their role in reimbursement of health care, the Medicare and Medicaid programs are important to health economics and outcomes research in several ways.

First, CMS and state agencies set coverage and reimbursement policies for the care provided to Medicare and Medicaid beneficiaries. Inasmuch as such policies affect the economic viability of health care products and services, producers of such products and services need to be able to justify their value in terms understandable to the relevant policymakers.

Second, Medicare and Medicaid public-use data can be analyzed to help understand the health care provided to beneficiaries of those programs and the associated costs. Burden (or cost) of illness studies are frequently performed using these data. However, one must be aware of the limitations as well as the advantages of using these data in such analyses. For example, inasmuch as Medicare does not cover prescription drugs, data on their use is not included in the public-use data. Additionally, little clinical detail is provided in the data. Medicaid data is also limited by the variability in program benefits across states and across time.

Enactment of the MPPPA came about because pharmaceuticals are the fastest growing cost in the Medicaid program, which typically accounts for between one-third and one-fifth of total state budget outlays. Despite its enactment, drug costs and health care costs continue to increase. This has led state legislatures to tighten eligibility, reduce benefits, or both. Such ongoing changes make it difficult to ascribe trends observed in analyses of Medicaid data to effective or ineffective care rather than to policy changes.

## ISSUES

The continuing increase of health care costs is an ongoing concern of policymakers responsible for the administration of the Medicare and Medicaid programs. While governments seek to contain costs, beneficiaries and health care providers request broader coverage of services and higher reimbursement levels respectively. The future form of these programs (e.g., who will be covered and for what and how much) will continue to be an ongoing debate.

## BIBLIOGRAPHY

Centers for Medicare and Medicaid Services (CMS). http://www.cms.gov/medicaid. Accessed March 31, 2003.
Medicare Web site. www.medicare.gov. Accessed March 31, 2003.

# Health Policy

## BRIEF DEFINITION

**Health policy** is the way that nations, states, cities, and communities distribute resources to competing interventions and competing populations based primarily on anticipated benefits. Health policy reflects the values of the society or community in terms of how and to whom health resources are distributed.

## EXPLANATION

Many factors can influence the health of populations including disease, injury, genetics, lifestyle, poverty, and stress, as well as the availability of adequate sanitation, clean water, and education. When health breaks down, many people turn (when available) to health care providers and institutions. Because resources are not infinite, the availability of and access to health care services are limited. Health policy reflects the values of the society or community in terms of how and to whom these scarce resources are distributed—based upon what is considered efficient (maximizing the benefit obtained), what is considered a minimally acceptable level of health care, and how resources can be equitably divided.

The process of developing health policy involves defining objectives and setting priorities. Monitoring and measuring the impact of health policy generally focuses on various aspects of health care delivery such as

- Setting and prioritizing objectives in health care
- Planning and financing health services
- Framing institutions to provide health care efficiently
- Organizing health care delivery
- Ensuring equity and access to health care, cost-effective production, and a combination of resources in health care
- Developing social health insurance
- Composing sophisticated health service packages

The instruments in health policy are health service programs designed to support the achievement of health policy objectives. For example, the World Health Organization in its struggle to reach the objectives of its "Health for All" initiative has designed programs to expand health infrastructures; to increase life expectancy; to improve nutrition, sanitation, and education; and to fight against infectious diseases, HIV/AIDS, and the abuse of tobacco. On a national level, health policy instruments are often regulations and incentives that enable or steer the provision of health services and access to those same services.

The formulation and design of health policy is a stepwise process:

1. Situation analysis: Definition of the key features or characteristics of population health and the health care system at a given time.
2. Objective formulation: Definition of objectives and indicators which allow the measurement of achievement.
3. Program design: Development of proper measures to achieve the objectives.
4. Program implementation.
5. Program evaluation: Appraisal of the measures taken to achieve the objectives and evaluation of the economic viability of these measures in comparison to standard care.

6. Program adaptation: If necessary after program evaluation using the insights from evaluation.

Health policy may take place at different levels of society and is driven by different stakeholders. From the governmental perspective, health policy takes place on a national, a regional (state), and a local level. With regard to health care delivery, physicians and their associations, hospitals and their associations, and other providers and their associations or unions try to shape health policy. On the payers' side, both public and private health insurances and other governmental or nongovernmental agencies and institutions try to influence health policy.

## VALUE AND USE

Health policy is an important part of social and economic policy that aims to promote the welfare and well-being of citizens of a nation or community. Health policy may also provide a framework for health economic analysis of health care processes and institutions in health care delivery. The term is often used as a surrogate for measures and legislation in health care or health care provision.

## ISSUES

Health policy offers a wide area of debate. Issues concerning system development are

- Determination of objectives and priorities
- Responsiveness to epidemiological realities and social needs
- Access for all members of society
- Centralized versus decentralized controlling of the health care system
- Systems and incentives to promote improvements of quality of health care
- Integration of medical innovation and progress
- Cost-effective health care
- Incentives to avoid wasting scarce resources
- Definition of basic packages of health care accessible for all and differentiation from additional health services to be purchased individually

Issues with regard to system behavior, processes (activities within the system), and health care delivery are

- Control of the process of health care delivery, i.e., the comprehensiveness and timeliness of process information
- The evidence of political measures for health
- Rising health care costs and cost containment
- The effectiveness of health care programs and measures
- The evaluation of policy recommendations in order to keep continuous improvement ongoing

BIBLIOGRAPHY

Abel-Smith B. *An Introduction to Health: Policy, Planning, Financing.* London: Longman; 1994.

Coast J, Donovan J, Frankel S. *Priority Setting: The Health Care Debate.* Chichester, UK: Wiley; 1996.

Mossialos E, Le Grand J. Health Care and Cost Containment in the European Union. Aldershot, UK: Ashgate; 1999.

Mossialos E, McKee M. Is a European healthcare policy emerging? *BMJ.* 2001;323:248.

Patrick D, Erickson P. *Health Status and Health Policy.* New York: Oxford University Press; 1993.

# Health-Related Quality of Life (HRQOL)

## BRIEF DEFINITION

**Health-related quality of life (HRQOL)** is a broad theoretical construct developed to explain and organize measures concerned with the evaluation of health status, attitudes, values, and perceived levels of satisfaction and general well-being with respect to either specific health conditions or life as a whole from the individual's perspective (*see term:* Patient-Reported Outcomes [PRO]).

## EXPLANATION

The definition of the term in the literature has shown a continuing lack of consensus about its conceptualization. Its very diffuseness and ambiguity is a reflection of its complex multidimensionality. The Patient-Reported Outcomes (PRO) Harmonization Group working in conjunction with the US Food and Drug Administration aimed to add clarity to the use of this term within the drug approval and labeling context by defining health-related quality of life as representing the patient's evaluation of the impact of a health condition and its treatment on daily life.

Despite difficulties in operationalizing the term, most measures of HRQOL include two or more of the following domains: physical functioning, social functioning, role functioning, mental health and general health, with concepts such as vitality (energy/fatigue), pain, and cognitive functioning subsumed under these broader categories.

These measures are generally based on one of two theoretical models. In the model that views domains as concentric circles, the innermost circle represents health characteristics that are intrinsic to the individual: disease, for example; and the outermost circle represents characteristics that are external to the individual: for example, social function. Instruments based on this model generate a profile of scores. The other model arrays health states, defined in terms of two or more domains, along a continuum that ranges from death to optimal health and incorporates preferences for health to form a summary measure of health.

Because many of the domains of HRQOL cannot be observed directly, HRQOL questionnaires are developed and evaluated according to the psychometric principles of test theory. This theory proposes that there is a true

HRQOL value that cannot be measured directly, but that can be measured indirectly by asking a series of questions (items). The answers to these questions are converted to numbers and combined to yield "scale scores," which may also be combined to yield domain scores or summary scores that are either statistically computed or preference-based. The resulting scale of measurement should differ from the corresponding true value of HRQOL only by random error of measurement and should possess several basic measurement properties (validity and reliability).

Another distinction between HRQOL instruments is whether they are generic or specific. Generic HRQOL instruments are designed to be applicable across all diseases or conditions, across different medical interventions and across a wide range of populations. In contrast, specific HRQOL measures are designed to be relevant to a particular health condition or population.

## VALUE AND USE

The debate about the inclusion of HRQOL when assessing the health outcomes of medical care has arisen in part from the challenge to previous outcomes, which have been predominantly conceptualized on the basis of epidemiological indicators of the presence or absence of disease and/or death (i.e., morbidity and mortality). Although it is true that these indicators are useful for depicting health outcomes of populations, the way health is understood and cared for has evolved toward providing more specific information on the health of defined individuals or groups. This transformation has to a large extent been caused by the numerous scientific and technical advances that have benefited medicine in recent decades and also by the improved living conditions in terms of housing, hygiene, and food. The application of the new medical knowledge along with the social and environmental improvements that have come about have increased patients' life expectancy and changed the patterns of morbidity away from highly lethal acute diseases to disabling chronic conditions.

While there is no single measure of HRQOL that has been found to be appropriate for use in all applications, there is general agreement that any measure of HRQOL should be designed to obtain self-report information from individuals in the target population. An individual's report of the impact of disease, treatment, or policy on symptoms, function, and perceptions, as well as treatment side effects and other health-related data, provide unique information. This information has been shown to be important for evaluating treatment efficacy and effectiveness and interpreting clinical outcomes as well as providing information about the benefits of alternative health interventions within the context of resource allocation.

## ISSUES

HRQOL reflects individuals' self-reports of health status and well-being collected from patients as well as members of the general population. With the continuing restricted state funding of welfare provision, HRQOL has been viewed as providing a standardized measure of "value for money," allowing the targeting of resources to areas that will achieve the best return from intervention.

## BIBLIOGRAPHY

Acquadro C, Berzon R, Dubois D, et al. Incorporating the patient's perspective into drug development and communication: An ad hoc task force report of the Patient-Reported Outcomes (PRO) Harmonization Group meeting of the Food and Drug Administration, February 16, 2001. *Value Health* 2003;6:522–531.

Leplège A, Hunt S. The problem of quality of life in medicine. *JAMA*. 1997;278:47–50.

Patrick DL, Erickson P. *Health Status and Health Policy: Quality of Life in Health Care Evaluation and Resource Allocation.* New York: Oxford University Press; 1993.

Rogerson RJ. Environmental and health-related quality of life: Conceptual and methodological similarities. *Soc Sci Med.* 1995;41:1373–1382.

Testa MA, Simonson DC. Assessment of quality of life outcomes. *N Eng J Med.* 1996;334:835–840.

# Health Status
Health
Mortality
Morbidity
Prognosis

## BRIEF DEFINITION
**Health status** can be defined as "functional capacity" or "a state of physiological and psychological functioning or well being." Health status has also been defined by the World Health Organization (WHO) as "the state of health of an individual, group or population measured against accepted standards." These standards would include the health expected of an individual of given age and medical condition.

## EXPLANATION
**Health** is a multidimensional construct that has been defined by the WHO as "a state of complete physical, mental and social well being, not merely the absence of disease or infirmity." Traditional measures of health have concentrated on mortality (quantity of life, followed by death) and morbidity (health-related quality of life). Since illness may both reduce life expectancy and render the remaining life less desirable, it has been deemed more appropriate to consider health status in terms of life expectancy (**mortality**), functioning and symptoms (**morbidity**), preference for a particular functional state (utility) (*see term:* Utility), and duration of stay in a particular health state (**prognosis**), according to the General Health Policy Model of Kaplan (1996) and others.

The primary aim of medical care is to improve or maintain the overall functional capacity and general health of patients, and medical care has traditionally concentrated on the diagnosis and treatment of physiological or anatomical conditions. More recent approaches have included patient self-reported global functioning, well-being, and quality of life. This has allowed for a more accurate assessment of individual or population health status and of the benefits and harms that may result from medical intervention.

## VALUE AND USE

There is no standard measure of health status, and observer assessment may include several dimensions such as the presence, absence, or risk of life threatening disease, severity of disease, and overall health. Individual health status may be elicited from a subject according to his or her health perceptions described in terms of physical functioning, emotional well-being, pain or discomfort, and overall perception of health. Subjective health status measurement can provide valuable data on the impact of clinical interventions on the daily lives of patients.

Health state measures have been advocated as the appropriate tools for the screening of patients requiring particular care. Normative data can be used to compare the health state of a particular patient group with that of the general population, while health status measures are now being routinely applied to cost utility studies to inform decisions on cost containment and prioritization of medical care.

## ISSUES

There remains some confusion over the measurement of health status and quality of life. Indeed, early measurements of quality of life used health status questionnaires that measured physical and psychological symptoms and other questionnaires designed to measure perceived distress, the impact of illness, physical functioning, and life satisfaction. The rationale for this was that aspects of life that were impacted by ill health must provide some insight into the impact on quality of life. This approach failed to recognize that subjective quality of life was more complex than mere assessment of physical, emotional, and social functioning. The results of a recent rigorous meta-analysis indicated that, from a patient perspective, quality of life and health status are clearly two distinct constructs. For example, mental health has a much greater impact on quality of life than physical functioning, while health status correlates more closely with perceived health.

## BIBLIOGRAPHY

Kaplan RM, Anderson JP. The general health policy model: An integrated approach. In: Spilker B, ed. *Quality of Life and Pharmacoeconomics in Clinical Trials*. New York: Raven; 1996.

Leplège A, Hunt S. The problem of quality of life in medicine. *JAMA*. 1997;278:47–50.

Murray CJL, Salomon JA, Mathers CD, Lopez AD. *Summary Measures of Population Health: Concepts, Ethics, Measurements, and Applications*. Geneva: World Health Organization; 2002.

Smith KW, Avis NE, Assmann SF. Distinguishing between quality of life and health status in quality of life research: a meta-analysis. *Qual Life Res*. 1999;8:447–459.

# Health Technology Assessment (HTA)
International Network of Health Technology Assessment Agencies (INAHTA)

## BRIEF DEFINITION

**Health technology assessment (HTA)** is a form of policy research that examines short- and long-term consequences of the application of a health care technology.

## EXPLANATION

The goal of HTA is to provide policymakers with information on policy alternatives. Health care technology within the concept of HTA is defined broadly as consisting of

- Drugs (e.g., aspirin, antibiotics, beta-blockers);
- Biologics (e.g., vaccines, blood products, biotechnology-derived substances);
- Devices, equipment, supplies (e.g., cardiac pacemaker, CT scanner, surgical gloves);
- Medical and surgical procedures (e.g., acupuncture, cancer chemotherapy, cesarean section);
- Support systems (e.g., drug formulary, clinical laboratory, patient record system); and
- Organizational, delivery, and managerial systems (e.g., emergency medical system, immunization program, disease management program, health care payment system).

For any given technology, properties and impacts assessed may include technical properties (this is particularly germane for sophisticated equipment), evidence of safety, efficacy (including patient-reported outcomes), real-world effectiveness, cost, and cost-effectiveness as well as estimated social, legal, ethical, and political impacts. Thus, HTA is conceived as being much broader than is typically true of health and economic outcomes research of a health care technology.

HTA is commonly performed at a national or multisystem level by governmental, quasi-governmental, or nonprofit organized groups and individuals to inform health care policies or decisions, such as to:

- Support decisions by industry about technology development and marketing,
- Advise regulatory agencies about allowing the marketing or use of a technology,
- Advise health plans and other payers concerning coverage and payment for a technology,
- Advise clinicians and patients about the appropriate use of a technology,
- Help managers of hospitals and other providers make decisions about acquiring a technology, and/or
- Support decisions by financial groups (e.g., venture capitalists) about investment in new technologies and companies.

## VALUE AND USE

In the broad sense depicted above, HTA can be (and is at times) employed by any person or groups. However, it was originally conceived as an adjunct to governmental policy decision making. This was exemplified by the US Congress's former Office of Technology Assessment, credited by many with having introduced HTA in a formal sense to United States society and indeed the world. Today, governments around the world have created internal agencies authorized to include a broad HTA function. The **International Network of Health Technology Assessment Agencies (INAHTA)** is an association of these governmental agencies. The respective governments look to these agencies to guide them in policy decisions such as those enumerated above.

There are also private HTA agencies, especially in the United States. Examples are Blue Cross Blue Shield's Technology Evaluation Center (TEC), ECRI, HAYES Inc, and the University HealthSystem Consortium. Although these private groups tend to practice a narrower brand of HTA than their public counterparts, their reports are viewed by their respective constituents as useful guidance for technology adoption and reimbursement decision making.

## ISSUES

A key issue associated with HTA, at least as it has been practiced at the governmental level (which has been its main focus worldwide) has been the lack of collaborative relationships between the innovators, producers, and advocates of health technology on the one hand and the governmental policymakers, on the other hand, who are the consumers of HTA and whose charge is to decide on societal adoption, use, and reimbursement of health care technologies.

## BIBLIOGRAPHY

Banta HD, Luce BR. Health Care Technology and its Assessment: An International Perspective. Oxford, UK: Oxford University Press, 1993.

# Health Utilities Index

## BRIEF DEFINITION

The **Health Utilities Index** (HUI™, Health Utilities Inc) is a generic, preference-scored system to measure health status, assess health-related quality of life, and produce utility scores.

## EXPLANATION

The HUI has two components. The first component is a multiattribute health status classification system that is used to describe health status. The second component is a multiattribute utility function that is used to value health status as measured by the first component. There are two systems, the HUI Mark II system (HUI2), and HUI Mark III system (HUI3). The only component that involves prospective primary data collection is the health status component. The health status component can be interview- or self-administered, involving self-assessment or proxy response. It is available in many languages.

The health status attributes included in the HUI systems are derived from a system first used in pediatrics, modified to become the current generic instruments. HUI2 utility scores are based on the preferences of a random sample of 293 parents of schoolchildren in Hamilton, Ontario. The utility scores for HUI3 are based on the preferences of 504 adults from Hamilton, Ontario. The utility scores, derived using a combination of visual analog scales and the standard gamble technique (*see term:* Utility Measurement), are based directly on von Neumann-Morgenstern utility theory and extensions to that theory to accommodate multiple attributes. Utility scores are available not only for the overall health state of the patient, but also for each attribute independently.

HUI2 consists of seven attributes: sensation (vision, hearing, speech), mobility, emotion, cognition, self-care, pain, and fertility. There are three to five levels per attribute, ranging from highly impaired to normal. Similarly, HUI3 consists of eight attributes: vision, hearing, speech, ambulation, dexterity, emotion, cognition, and pain. There are five to six levels per attribute. HUI2 defines 24,000 unique health states, HUI3 defines 972,000. The system has been used in a wide variety of clinical areas and many different countries. Reliability, validity, and responsiveness have been demonstrated in many different applications. For further details see the Web site http://www.healthutilities.com.

## Value and Use

The HUI systems are used to document health status, to quantify health-related quality of life in utility units, to provide the utilities needed to calculate quality-adjusted life years for use in cost-utility analysis (*see term:* Cost-Utility Analysis), and to quantify and compare population health. An HUI questionnaire takes a few minutes for completion if interviewer-administered and from 5 to 10 minutes if self-administered.

There is overlap between HUI2 and HUI3; however, in some ways, the two systems complement each other. For example, the concepts of emotion differ between the two systems: HUI2 refers to worry and anxiety while HUI3 to happiness versus depression. Similarly, the concepts of pain differ: while both refer to the degree of severity of the pain, HUI2 focuses on the use of analgesia while HUI3 focuses on the disruption of activities. Self-care and fertility are addressed only in HUI2; dexterity is addressed only in HUI3. HUI2 has been extensively used in clinical studies, providing useful benchmark results for comparisons. HUI3 has been used in four major Canadian population health surveys, providing extensive data on population norms. It has been shown through practice that in clinical studies, the two complement each other in substantial ways.

## Issues

Both HUI2 and HUI3 focus on a person's physical capacity rather than his or her actual performance, although in some instances, such as when a proxy respondent is used, observed performance stands as the indication of capacity. Both also adopt a "within the skin" definition of health status, focusing on physical and emotional dimensions of health, excluding social interaction.

Both HUI2 and HUI3 were scored using Canadian subjects. Are these utility scores appropriate in other countries? Evidence suggests they are. HUI3 scoring has been replicated in France with very similar results. This is consistent with the bulk of the utility literature that finds that geographic location of respondent is not a significant determinant of utility score.

BIBLIOGRAPHY

Feeny D, Furlong W, Torrance GW, et al. Multiattribute and single-attribute utility functions for the Health Utilities Index Mark 3 system. *Med Care.* 2002;40:113–128.

Feeny DH, Torrance GW, Furlong WJ. Health Utilities Index. In: Spilker B, ed. *Quality of Life and Pharmacoeconomics in Clinical Trials.* Philadelphia: Lippincott-Raven; 1996.

Furlong WJ, Feeny DH, Torrance GW, Barr RD. The health utilities index (HUI) system for assessing health-related quality of life in clinical studies. *Ann Med.* 2001;33:375–384.

# Healthy-Years Equivalent (HYE)

## BRIEF DEFINITION

**Healthy-years equivalent** (HYE) is a health outcome measure that combines preferences for quality of life and quantity of life into a single metric. It is the hypothetical number of years spent in good health that is considered equivalent to the actual number of years spent in a defined imperfect state of health or in a series of defined imperfect states of health.

## EXPLANATION

Healthy-years equivalent (HYE) is in a group of outcome measures that combine quality of life and quantity of life into a single number. Unlike the more commonly used approach to determining quality-adjusted life years (QALY) (*see term:* Quality-Adjusted Life Year [QALY]), which measures preferences for each single health state separately and combines these preferences, the HYE approach measures the preference for the whole sequence of health states simultaneously. This means the HYE more properly accounts for preferences associated with the timing and sequencing aspects of the health states. However, it also means that each measurement is much more complicated and that many more measurements are needed. Each different time sequence of health states (different durations or different order) requires its own measurement.

The HYE for each different time sequence of health states is determined by a two-stage standard gamble (*see term:* Utility Measurement) measurement procedure. In the first stage, a standard gamble is used to determine the conventional utility of the time sequence of health states. In the second stage, another standard gamble is used to determine the number of healthy years that would give the same utility. Interestingly, these two standard gambles used in this way are equivalent to a single time trade-off (*see term:* Utility Measurement) procedure and in practice would differ only by measurement error.

## Issues

The first stage in the HYE measurement provides a better utility for a time sequence of health states than the conventional approach of measuring the utility of each state singly and combining over time. However, in most studies the improvement comes with a dramatic increase in measurement burden. It remains to be seen whether the increase in accuracy is sufficient to justify the additional burden.

The second stage produces the actual HYE. However, an HYE is not a utility and is not intended as an alternative to utility theory. It is intended as a useful communication tool for those not comfortable with utilities and decision trees. If one desires an HYE, it is simpler to use the single stage time trade-off approach rather than the two-stage standard gamble approach.

## Bibliography

Gafni A. HYEs: Do we need them and can they fulfill the promise? *Med Dec Making.* 1996;16:215–216.

Mehrez A, Gafni A. The healthy-years equivalents: how to measure them using the standard gamble approach. *Med Decis Making.* 1991;11:140–146.

Wakker P. A criticism of healthy-years equivalents. *Med Decis Making.* 1996;16:207–214.

# Incidence
Incidence Rate
Cumulative Incidence
Incidence Density
Hazard Rate

BRIEF DEFINITION
Incidence is the frequency of *new* cases of an event that develop within a given time period in a defined population at risk.

EXPLANATION
Incidence quantifies the number of new cases or events that develop in a defined population at risk during a given time period. Traditionally, the "event" has been the occurrence of disease, but incidence can also be used for occurrence of any health-related event such as death, side effects, disease remission, or admission to a hospital.

There are two main ways to consider an **incidence rate: cumulative incidence** and **incidence density**. Cumulative incidence is calculated with the denominator representing the number of individuals. In incidence density, the corresponding person-years at risk among members of the source population is placed in the denominator. An incidence rate or density can be used to estimate a **hazard rate**.

$$\text{Cumulative Incidence} = \frac{\text{Number of new cases in a given time period}}{\text{Number of persons at risk in the same time period}}$$

$$\text{Incidence Density} = \frac{\text{Number of new cases in a given time period}}{\text{Number of person-years of risk in the population}}$$

VALUE AND USE
Incidence rates are used to estimate probability of occurrence or the risk of an event. Incidence rates for groups with certain characteristics (e.g., exposed and nonexposed) are compared and relative risks are calculated. Incidences are also used to measure morbidity in the population. From a public health point of view, it is important to follow changes in incidence for various diseases, such as, for example, cancer diseases over time.

Cumulative incidence is most widely used for cohort (longitudinal) studies in which the same group of people is followed over time. Incidence density is used in the situation of an ever-changing population (e.g., in an open-enrollment clinical trial where patients are followed for different lengths of time) or when exposure time varies among those under study (e.g., occupational exposure or drug exposure).

There is an interrelationship between incidence (I), prevalence (P), and the average duration of the disease (D) in a stable situation and assuming that the prevalence of the disease in the population is low—that is, less than 0.1.

$$P = I \times D$$

ISSUES

The numerator of an incidence rate is the number of new cases within a time period. The time period chosen should be long enough to ensure a stable measure. The denominator of the incidence rate should reflect the number of persons at risk or under study for the event. The denominator should exclude individuals who already have or already had the event of interest, unless recurrence is possible, such as the case with side effects or admission to a hospital. However, in large population studies, such as using census data, the denominator is usually not corrected for individuals who currently have or had the event of interest.

BIBLIOGRAPHY

Hennekens CH, Buring JE. *Epidemiology in medicine.* Boston: Little, Brown and Company; 1987.

Lilienfeld DE, Stolley PD. *Foundations of epidemiology.* New York: Oxford University Press; 1994.

Morton RF, Hebel JR, McCarter RJ. *A study guide to epidemiology and biostatistics.* Gaithersburg, Md: Aspen Publishers; 1996.

Timmreck TC. *An introduction to epidemiology.* Boston: Jones and Bartlett Publisher; 1994.

# Influence Diagram

BRIEF DEFINITION

An **influence diagram**, like a decision tree (*see term:* Decision Tree), are representations of the logical structure of a decision; they can be used both to visually communicate the elements of a problem and to assist in conducting quantitative decision analysis (*see term:* Decision Analysis).

EXPLANATION

An influence diagram is a model constructed using symbols ("nodes") to represent each decision and to represent uncertainty that may influence the outcome of a process. Connecting arrows, referred to as arcs of influence, indicate relationships among the nodes, such as conditional probabilities or other values or time ordering.

Influence diagrams may be considered structural alternatives to decision trees, as they are mathematically equivalent.

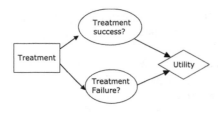

## VALUE AND USE

Influence diagrams are used to graphically depict a problem, including all factors that have an impact on the outcome of a given decision or process. They have some of the same uses in decision analysis as decision trees. Like decision (or probability) trees, influence diagrams depict the decisions, chance events, and objectives that define the problem. Unlike decision trees, however, an influence diagram does not depict the alternative actions for a decision or all the possible outcomes of each event. This results in a less comprehensive, but much more compact representation of the same model. Influence diagrams also have the advantage of explicitly showing the influencing relationships between factors (decisions, events, parameters).

## ISSUES

If the influence diagram is used analytically, the modeler/analyst faces the same challenges as when using decision trees and other types of models. Specifically, the output derived from the model depends on the accuracy and comprehensiveness of the data inputs.

Also, because influence diagrams do not comprehensively display the alternatives of decisions or the outcomes of events, they have the disadvantage, relative to decision trees, of not being able to display the complete set of relationships at a particular decision point. Further, they are not typically able to show asymmetry—situations in which some events or alternatives may not occur in all paths.

## BIBLIOGRAPHY

Clemen RT. *Making Hard Decisions: An Introduction to Decision Analysis.* 2nd ed. Belmont, Calif: Wadsworth Publishing Co.; 1996.

Nease RF Jr, Owens DK. Use of influence diagrams to structure medical decisions. *Med Decis Making.* 1997;17:263–275.

Owens DK, Shachter RD, Nease RF Jr. Representation and analysis of medical decision problems with influence diagrams. *Med Decis Making.* 1997;17:351–352.

# Labeling
Label
Misbranding
Off-Label

## BRIEF DEFINITION
According to the Medical Subject Headings (MeSH) definition, drug **labeling** is the use of written, printed, graphic materials upon or accompanying a drug container or wrapper. It includes contents, indications, effects, dosages, routes, methods, frequency and duration of administration, warnings, hazards, contraindications, side effects, precautions, and other relevant information.

According to the MeSH definition, food labeling is the use of written, printed, graphic materials upon or accompanying a food container or wrapper. The concept includes ingredients, nutritional value, directions, warnings, and other relevant information.

## EXPLANATION
In the United States, regulations for labeling are decided by the Food and Drug Administration (FDA) (*see term:* Food and Drug Administration [FDA]). Since the early 1960s, the FDA has required that drugs used in the United States be both safe and effective. The label information—on the container, in the package insert, in the Physicians Desk Reference (PDR), and in any advertising—can indicate a drug's use only in certain "approved" doses and routes of administration for a particular condition. The 1962 revision of the law spelled out strict new procedures for drug clearance, recording and reporting experience with new drugs, drug labeling, factory inspection, drug manufacturing controls, drug patents, and control of information and drug advertising to physicians. Labeling provides information on a drug, food, device, or cosmetic to the purchaser or user.

**Label** refers to a sign on the container, adhesive label, a package insert, a reference text, or any other physical bearer of information regulating the use of the product. The label must contain directions for use (unless exempted by regulation) and warnings. It may not contain false or misleading information.

Improper and/or illegal labeling of a drug or drug product as a consequence of incomplete disclosure of material facts and/or misleading inaccurate wording is known as **misbranding**.

The use of a drug for a disease not listed on the label or in a dose or by a route not listed on the label is considered to be a "nonapproved" or "unlabel" or off-label use of the drug. The FDA policies on off-label use restrict proactive distribution of written materials and discussions of off-label uses by pharmaceutical manufacturers or other manufacturers of medical products. Any other party without a financial interest is allowed to discuss off-label uses.

## VALUE AND USE

Labeling information is derived from the New Drug Application (NDA) that the FDA reviews in order to determine whether a drug may be marketed in the United States. The label may be revised as additional important information becomes available about the risks and benefits of the drug for approved indications. The data that are reflected in labeling encompass such aspects as clinical pharmacology (mechanism of action and pharmacokinetics), indications and uses, dosages for different types of patients, available forms of therapy, contraindications, precautions, side effects and adverse reactions, special considerations, patient and family education, and monitoring parameters. The developed information is meant for health professionals, and it explains the efficacy of a drug and alerts practitioners to certain dangers and restrictions in its use. The FDA regulations of labeling ensure a high standard of safety and efficacy of marketed drugs.

## ISSUES

Physicians, based on their knowledge and on available current information, may use a drug for a use not indicated in the "approved" labeling if it seems reasonable or appropriate. With the rising costs of health care and the desire to curb these costs, the issue of coverage and reimbursement for the "off-label" use of drugs has become an issue.

Eighty percent of drugs referenced in PDR are not labeled for use in children. An extremely large number of off-label uses is characteristic in the areas of pediatrics, oncology, and HIV. Recent actions by legislative bodies, the FDA, and the National Institutes of Health offer remedial measures to increase development of data to support labeling of drugs for pediatric and oncology indications.

## BIBLIOGRAPHY

Brian J. Using the Web for label approval. Web-based label proofreading can cut the time it takes to initiate a global trial. *Applied Clinical Trials*. 1999;8:54.

Halvorsen RL, Iacobucci JG. Current clinical labeling concepts: An introduction. *Applied Clinical Trials*. 1992;1:48.

Hölzer AW. Integrated labeling for randomized clinical trials. *Applied Clinical Trials*. 1993;2:62.

Mascaro J, Korteweg M. Investigational medicinal product labeling in Europe. *Applied Clinical Trials*. 1993;2:44.

Moult AN, Noblet M. Meeting multilingual label requirements for clinical trials materials. *Applied Clinical Trials*. 2000;9:E3.

Rogers LC, Cocchetto DM. Labeling prescription drugs for pediatric use in the United States. *Applied Clinical Trials*. 1997;6:50.

Wechsler J. Regulating off-label information on the internet. *Applied Clinical Trials*. 1997;6:14.

# Likelihood Ratio
## Receiver Operating Characteristic (ROC) Curve

### BRIEF DEFINITION

**Likelihood ratio** is a statistical test used to determine how many times more (or less) likely a diagnostic test result is to be found in diseased, as compared to nondiseased, people (*see term:* Predictive Value). For a positive test, the likelihood ratio is the odds of the sensitivity versus the false-positive rate, which is equal to sensitivity/(1 − specificity). In diagnostic testing, this is the ratio of true-positives to false-positives.

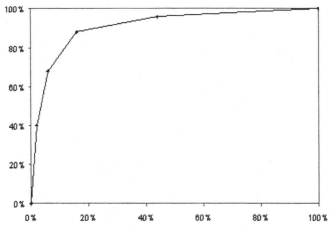

A ROC curve plots the false positive rate on the X-axis and 1 minus the false negative rate on the Y-axis. It shows the trade-off between the two rates. If the area under the ROC curve is close to 1, you have a very good test result; if the area is close to 0.5, you have a very bad test result.

### EXPLANATION

Likelihood ratios are useful in determining a diagnostic test's accuracy in identifying people with the target disorder. Two questions need to be answered in order to obtain a likelihood ratio: how likely it is to get a given test result among people with the target disorder and how likely it is to get the same test result among people without the target disorder. The likelihood ratio indicates by how much a given diagnostic test result will raise or lower the pretest probability of the target disorder. This can also be displayed graphically using a **receiver operating characteristic (ROC) curve** (see figure). An ROC curve can be used to display this relationship visually for a diagnostic test with a continuous outcome and arbitrary cut point. This curve expresses the sensitivity (the correct signal) and the false positive rate (the noise) for a given test. The true positives (sensitivity) are plotted on the Y-axis and the false-positives are plotted on the X-axis. The resulting curve helps to evaluate the properties (sensitivity, specificity, and accuracy) of the diagnostic test. On an ROC curve, the closer to the upper left-hand corner the curve is, the more accurate are the results of the test because the true positive rate is approaching 1 and the false-positive rate is approaching 0. As the sensitivity and specificity of a given test change, the corresponding point on the ROC curve will change. The area under the ROC curve indicates the accuracy of the test, with a value of 1 representing 100 percent sensitivity and specificity and a value of 0.5 representing no discriminatory power. An ROC curve is a graphical representation of the trade-off between the false negative and false positive rates for every possible cut-off. By tradition, the plot shows the false positive rate on the X-axis and 1 minus the false negative rate on the Y-axis.

## VALUE AND USE

In diagnostic testing, the likelihood ratio is used to convert a physician's pretest probability that the patient is diseased to the posttest probability of the patient's disease status based on the diagnostic test properties. This is accomplished by converting pretest probabilities into odds (probability disease/[1 − probability disease]), multiplying by the likelihood ratio (property of the diagnostic test), and converting the posttest odds into a posttest probability (odds/[odds + 1]).

## ISSUES

While calculating likelihood ratios and interpreting ROC curves is not difficult, recent studies of physician frequency of using these methods to appraise a test's diagnostic accuracy are not good. Physicians cited nonfamiliarity with likelihood ratios and ROC curves as the main reason they did not use them and retreated back to determining how often a test was right or wrong in patients who later became diseased and nondiseased. Whether this technique is valid is still being investigated.

## BIBLIOGRAPHY

Dawson-Saunders B, Trapp RG. *Basic and Clinical Biostatistics.* 2nd ed. Norwalk, Conn: Appleton and Lange; 1994.

Jaeschke R, Guyatt GH, Sackett DL. Users' guide to the medical literature: III. How to use an article about a diagnostic test; B. What are the results and will they help me in caring for my patients? *JAMA.* 1994;27:703–707.

Reid MC, Lane DA, Feinstein AR. Academic calculations versus clinical judgments: practicing physicians' use of quantitative measures of test accuracy. *Am J Med.* 1998;104:374–380.

# Literature Overview
## Literature Review
## Systematic Review
## Meta-Analysis

## BRIEF DEFINITION

A **literature overview** can be any of the three types of literature summarization of a specific topic. A **literature review** is a nonquantitative summary of existing published literature. A **systematic review**, also known as a structured literature review, is similar in that it summarizes a topic, but it does so in a systematic fashion using preset criteria and a protocol. **Meta-analysis** is both a systematic literature review and a quantitative synthesis of findings across multiple studies.

## EXPLANATION

A literature review is a type of study generally performed to provide a (relatively) brief overview of the published literature in a specified area. The review allows readers to become familiar with a large body of work that they are unlikely to read comprehensively themselves. Reviews can summarize literature in a particular clinical area, studies using a specific type of methodology, or other common themes. Information is often presented in both text and table formats. Literature reviews (as distinct from systematic reviews) tend not to summarize quantitatively a body of literature or set of findings. However, literature reviews may provide subjective conclusions regarding the included studies.

A systematic review has two major features that distinguish it from a traditional literature review. First, there is a formal and comprehensive search for relevant literature. This generally includes searching computerized literature databases such as MEDLINE and EMBASE plus all other pertinent databases for all relevant studies (as identified by selected keywords). Additional relevant studies may be found from references in identified literature or by discussions with experts in the field being reviewed. Second, there are explicit, objective criteria for selecting studies to be included. That is, only studies meeting certain criteria (inclusion and/or exclusion criteria) will be accepted for the review. These criteria are generally set, prior to the initiation of the systematic search, in a transparent manner for use by all potential reviewers. Both the search strategy and inclusion/exclusion criteria should be specified in a systematic literature review. Systematic literature reviews may also evaluate the quality of reviewed literature.

Meta-analysis involves both a systematic review and a quantitative combination of results across similar studies. Evaluation of potential studies and abstraction of data from included studies may be performed by multiple independent reviewers to decrease the risk of bias. Multiple reviewers using various scoring instruments usually assess the quality of all articles. In addition, funnel plots may be created to summarize results and inspect for potential publication bias.

Meta-analysis is generally performed on published studies but may also include unpublished studies. Inclusion of unpublished studies may decrease the quality of the meta-analysis, as results from such studies have not been subject to the peer review process. However, unpublished studies may have more recent findings than do published studies. Further, to the extent that there is a publication bias against studies with negative findings, unpublished studies may be more likely to have negative information. Thus, inclusion of unpublished studies may or may not improve the overall accuracy of the meta-analysis.

Following systematic literature review and selection, study findings are combined to produce quantitative summary results. The meta-analysis methodology for combining studies can involve either "fixed effects" or "random effects." Briefly, "fixed effects" indicates that the results of the analysis are conditional on the populations of the included studies, while "random effects" assumes that the study results reflect outcomes in a broader population.

## VALUE AND USE

In addition to summarizing succinctly a body of work, literature reviews also provide primary references that can be examined for more detailed information. They thus facilitate the rapid familiarization of readers with a set of studies.

Systematic reviews provide a more objective summary of a body of literature than do traditional literature reviews. They are more likely to discuss all relevant literature within a given area and are thus less likely to be influenced by article selection bias. However, conclusions from the discussed literature are still subjective and are subject to reviewer (or other) bias.

Meta-analyses are typically used to increase the statistical power available to assess an intervention's effect on key outcomes and to better understand the size of that effect as well as to assess the outcome effect on subcohorts. Results of meta-analysis can be used to assess the effectiveness of a health care product or service or to plan new studies, especially in those cases where the existing literature is composed primarily of studies with small cohort sizes and conflicting results. Meta-analyses provide the most quantitatively accurate summary of a body of literature.

## ISSUES

In a traditional literature review, there is generally no systematic method used to identify or include studies. Rather, reviewers focus on literature that they consider to be representative of the overall field of work or importance, or that is readily accessible or familiar to them. Inclusion of particular studies in a literature review is therefore highly subjective, and the review may be biased. Self-quotation is widespread.

While the literature identification and inclusion process in a systematic literature review is objective, findings from included studies may not always be combined in a quantitative fashion across studies. Overall characteristics of the included studies, such as the number of studies showing a positive effect of a particular therapy, may be quantified.

Meta-analysis has traditionally been used to combine data on clinical outcomes (e.g., efficacy, mortality, adverse event rates) across studies. However, the methodology can be used to combine economic or quality of life outcomes across studies in a robust manner. Study quality can also be incorporated into a meta-analysis by using an objective (and predefined) quality scoring system and stratifying studies based on their score. Such quality scores may, nonetheless, include subjective elements and value judgments. Unfortunately, the underlying studies in a particular therapeutic area or the studies that are available to answer a specific therapeutic question may not be sufficiently comparable to permit a meta-analysis to be performed.

In all overviews, the quality of the output is directly dependent upon the quality of inputs. A pertinent issue when examining the quality of the literature is that reviewers are never certain whether they are measuring the quality of the research that has been done or the quality of the writing of the manuscript. Another issue is the ability to detect original research and separate it from duplicate or overlapping studies. Often, one paper may appear in many forms, sometimes as verbatim copies (i.e., redundant publications), with minor modifications (e.g., adding a few new cases, but with essentially the same results), or as the same study with a different outcome.

## BIBLIOGRAPHY

Laird NM, Mostellar F. Some statistical methods for combining experimental results. *Int J Technol Assess Health Care.* 1990;6:5–30.

Mulrow CD. Rationale for systematic reviews. *BMJ.* 1994;309:597–599.

Oxman AD, Guyatt GH. Guidelines for reading literature reviews. *CMAJ.* 1988;138:697–703.

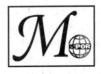

# Managed Care Organization (MCO)
Health Maintenance Organization (HMO)
Staff Model HMO
Group Model HMO
Network HMO
Independent Practice Association (IPA)
Preferred Provider Organization (PPO)

## BRIEF DEFINITION
Any entity that utilizes managed care concepts or techniques to manage the accessibility, cost, and quality of health care in the provision of health care benefits to eligible populations is considered a **managed care organization (MCO)**.

## EXPLANATION
Managed care organizations are entities that manage the use of medical services and the attendant costs of services within the MCO and that measure the process and quality of health care delivery. The goal is a system that delivers value by giving people access to high quality, cost-effective health care.

Managed care has grown out of the original concept of prepaid health care. In managed care, individuals who pay a certain amount of money each month are eligible to receive a package of health benefits with no appreciable extra charge. The MCOs try to market competitively the best benefits for the lowest prices to their members. Typically managed care organizations exchange lower plan costs for tighter control of the process by which a patient can use medical services.

Managed care organizations generally share the following hallmarks: integration of financing and management with the delivery of health care services to an enrolled population; employment of or contracting with an organized provider network that delivers services and which, as a network or individual provider, either shares financial risk or has some incentives to deliver high quality, cost-effective services; use of an information system capable of monitoring and evaluating the patterns of covered persons' use of medical services and the cost and quality of those services.

Managed care organizations may provide services to self-enrolled individuals, employees of companies, and government-enrolled persons (Medicare and Medicaid beneficiaries).

The term "managed care organization" generally includes, but is not limited to, the following:

**Health maintenance organization (HMO).** A licensed health plan that places some medical risk, either directly or indirectly, on providers. These plans typically provide a capitated payment to providers on a per-member per-month basis. These organizations do not typically cover services provided out of a predefined network of providers.

**Staff model HMO.** An HMO in which the physicians are salaried full-time employees who provide services exclusively to the HMO enrollees. Providers typically share no direct financial risk with the HMO, although they are subject to utilization reviews.

**Group model HMO.** An HMO that contracts with a multispecialty group practice that provides services exclusively to the HMO enrollees. Unlike staff model HMOs, group model HMOs bear some direct financial risk.

**Network HMO.** An HMO that contracts with two or more group practices but does not require the practices to provide exclusive care to the HMO enrollees. Network HMOs operate under direct risk sharing arrangements but are also able to provide care to patients outside the HMO.

**Independent practice association (IPA).** IPAs contract with multiple solo and small group practices on a nonexclusive basis. IPA HMOs utilize capitation and other direct risk sharing arrangements with differing degrees of success. IPAs typically have very little control over physician practices, as the majority of the providers' business tends to be outside the HMO.

**Preferred provider organization (PPO).** In a PPO, a plan's members are allowed to seek care from a physician of their choosing, but they have significant financial incentives to seek care from a list of providers compiled by the managed care organization. Providers are not capitated; rather, they provide services at a discounted fee-for-service rate in exchange for a higher volume of patients.

## VALUE AND USE

Managed care organizations and practices are generally believed to contribute to lower overall medical costs and improved patient care.

## ISSUES

The cost, quality, and access to health care remains a significant societal concern, and the role of managed care continues to evolve. Managed care organizations continue to struggle with negative perceptions among consumers and relationships with providers.

## BIBLIOGRAPHY

American Association of Health Plans. http://www.aahp.org/glossary/index.html. Accessed January 14, 2003.

Kongstvedt PR. *Essentials of Managed Health Care.* 2nd ed. Washington, DC: Aspen Publications; 1973.

Navarro R, Wertheimer AI. *Managing the Pharmacy Benefit.* Wayne, NJ: Emron Publishing; 1996.

Rakich JS, Longest BB. *Managing Health Services Organizations.* 3rd ed. Baltimore: Health Professions Press; 1992.

Sultz HA, Young KM. *Healthcare USA, Understanding its Organization and Delivery.* Gaithersburg, Md: Aspen Publications; 1997.

Wan TH. *Analysis and Evaluation of Health Care Systems—An Integrated Approach to Managerial Decision Making.* Baltimore, MD: Health Professions Press; 1995.

# Medical Device

## BRIEF DEFINITION

A **medical device** is any instrument, apparatus, appliance, or related article that is intended for use in the diagnosis, prevention, monitoring, treatment, or alleviation of disease or that is intended to affect the structure or function of the human anatomy. A medical device may not achieve its principal intended action through pharmacological, immunological, or metabolic means. Examples of medical devices include cardiac balloon catheters and coronary stents (including drug-coated stents), endoscopes, magnetic resonance imaging machines, artificial hip joints, etc.

## EXPLANATION

The medical device definition is derived from the need of government bodies to regulate marketing of these products and for payers to cover and pay for them. In the United States, the Food and Drug Administration (FDA) regulates the pre- and postmarketing of medical devices. The FDA defines a medical device as

> An instrument, apparatus, implement, machine, contrivance, implant, in vitro reagent, or other similar or related article, including a component part, or accessory which is:
> - Recognized in the official National Formulary, or the United States Pharmacopoeia, or any supplement to them,
> - Intended for use in the diagnosis of disease or other conditions, or in the cure, mitigation, treatment, or prevention of disease, in man or other animals, or
> - Intended to affect the structure or any function of the body of man or other animals, and which does not achieve any of its primary intended purposes through chemical action within or on the body of man or other animals and which is not dependent upon being metabolized for the achievement of any of its primary intended purposes.

Three European directives regulate all medical devices in the European Union. The directive that defines a medical device is as follows:

> Any instrument, apparatus, appliance, material or other article, whether used alone or in combination, including the software necessary for its proper application intended by the manufacturer to be used for human beings for the purpose of:
> - Diagnosis, prevention, monitoring, treatment or alleviation of disease,

- Diagnosis, monitoring, treatment, alleviation of or compensation for an injury or handicap,
- Investigation, replacement or modification of the anatomy or of a physiological process,
- Control of conception,
- And which does not achieve its principal intended action in or on the human body by pharmacological, immunological or metabolic means, but which may be assisted in its function by such means.

The medical device regulatory bodies of other countries have similar definitions.

## ISSUES

Often, medical device definitions may differ between government regulations and payer coverage and payment criteria. For example, the Medicare Program in the United States has a medical device definition for coverage and payment that is different from the FDA definition. Medicare covers durable medical equipment, supplies, and prosthetic devices. Medicare defines durable medical equipment as equipment that

- Can withstand repeated use; i.e., could normally be rented, and used by successive patients;
- Is primarily and customarily used to serve a medical purpose;
- Generally is not useful to a person in the absence of illness or injury; and
- Is appropriate for use in a patient's home.

Medicare states that supplies and accessories as

- Are necessary for the effective use of durable medical equipment (e.g., oxygen).
- Such supplies include those drugs and biologicals which must be put directly into the equipment in order to achieve the therapeutic benefit of the durable medical equipment or to assure the proper functioning of the equipment, e.g., tumor chemotherapy agents used with an infusion pump or heparin used with a home dialysis system.

Prosthetic devices, according to Medicare

- Replace all or part of an internal body organ (including contiguous tissue), or
- Replace all or part of the function of a permanently inoperative or malfunctioning internal body organ.
- Examples of prosthetic devices include cardiac pacemakers, prosthetic lenses, breast prostheses (including a surgical brassiere) for post-mastectomy patients, maxillofacial devices and devices which replace all or part of the ear or nose. A urinary collection and retention system with or without a tube is a prosthetic device replacing bladder function in case of permanent urinary incontinence. The Foley catheter is also considered a prosthetic device when ordered for a patient with permanent urinary incontinence.

Among other supplies, appliances, and devices, Medicare includes

- Surgical dressings, and splints, casts, and other devices used for reduction of fractures and dislocations.

The new ICD-10 procedure coding system, which may be implemented by the Center for Medicare and Medicaid Services (CMS) and other payers in the near future, has a different definition of medical device for coding purposes.

The term "device" is used to specify only devices that remain after the procedure is completed. Instruments that describe how a procedure is performed are not specified in the device character. Materials that are incidental to a procedure such as clips and sutures are not considered devices.
- Biological or synthetic material that takes the place of all or a portion of a body part (e.g., skin grafts and joint prostheses)
- Biological or synthetic material that assists or prevents a physiological function (e.g., IUD).
- Therapeutic material that is not absorbed by, eliminated by, or incorporated into a body part (e.g., radioactive implant). Therapeutic materials that are considered devices can always be removed.
- Mechanical or electronic appliances used to assist, monitor, take the place of, or prevent a physiological function (e.g., diaphragmatic pacemaker, orthopedic pins).
- Examples include: drainage device, radioactive element, autograft, extraluminal device, intraluminal device, synthetic substitute, tissue substitute

BIBLIOGRAPHY

International Classification of Diseases. 10th ed. Baltimore: Center for Medicare and Medicaid Services; 1998.

Food, Drug and Cosmetic Act, 21 CFR §201(h), parts 800–1299 (1998).

Medical Device Directive, Council Directive 93/42/EEC of 14 June 1993 concerning medical devices, 1–46.

US Department of Health and Human Services Centers for Medicare & Medicaid Services. *Medicare Coverage Issues Manual.* Section 60-11. November 29, 2002, and Medicare Intermediary Manual, Part 3, Chapter VII–Bill Review. http://www.cms/hhs.gov/manuals/13_int/a3676.asp. Accessed September 25, 2003.

# Modeling

| | |
|---|---|
| Monte Carlo Simulation | Evidence Model |
| Deterministic Analysis | Probabilistic Sensitivity Analysis |
| Treatment Model | Stochastic Sensitivity Analysis |
| Markov Model | |

BRIEF DEFINITION

**Modeling** refers to the development of a simplified representation of a system (e.g., a population). A particular model may be analytical, visual, or both. In pharmacoeconomics specifically or health economics in general, analytical models can be used to pose and answer questions about interventions that cannot be directly answered by clinical trials due to time and financial constraints (*see terms:* Health Economics, Pharmacoeconomics).

**Monte Carlo simulation** refers to the use of a computer to repeatedly evaluate a model, usually to quantify either the level of confidence in recommendations based on the model (a form of sensitivity analysis) (*see term:* Sensitivity Analysis), or the level of risk associated with an intervention.

EXPLANATION

Models can be

- Analytical—a mathematical or statistical representation of reality, with intermediate and/or final "outputs" (e.g., life expectancy) that respond to changes in "inputs" (e.g., particular risk factors) in a realistic way; and
- Visual—use symbols to represent key events, temporal and/or causal relationships and dependencies, and outcomes.

A variety of dedicated software packages, spreadsheet plug-ins, and even specialized software languages can be used in constructing simple and complex analytical and visual models.

Decision trees (*see term:* Decision Tree) (and related probability trees) are a common form of health economics model that can have both analytical and

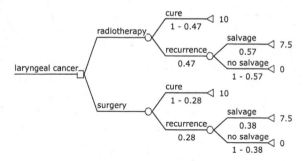

Example of a decision tree

visual aspects. An influence diagram (*see term:* Influence Diagram) and flow charts are often used as purely visual models, while models built in spreadsheets are often analytical only.

**Deterministic analysis** is a standard method of evaluation used with analytical models in which, for a specified set of inputs (even inputs randomly drawn from probability distributions), the model will always return the same result. Model results can then be used in decision analysis or cost-effectiveness analysis.

Some methods exist for automated construction of predictive analytical models from data sets (e.g., neural network algorithms, multivariate regression models). However, modeling often involves attention to the nuances of what is being modeled and, therefore, customization of each model structure to pro-

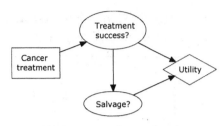

Example of an influence diagram

mote accuracy and to ensure an optimal trade-off between interpretability and comprehensiveness. This is especially true of a complex health economics **treatment model**, such as a **Markov model**, that describe the natural history of particular diseases, with and without treatment. To capture all critical events, Markov models can categorize health status with a higher level of detail and divide the model's time perspective into finer intervals than is possible with decision trees.

Data availability and quality issues are of crucial importance in pharmacoeconomic modeling. The model builder often must synthesize clinical data and other information from multiple sources. The evidence search can be guided by an **evidence model**—a set of precise statements describing such issues as (1) relationships between the clinical decisions or intervention(s) and health outcomes, (2) the health providers responsible for the decisions or intervention(s), and (3) the target patient population. If the evidence search finds disagreement in estimates of crucial model parameters, meta-analysis can sometimes be used to reconcile them. Simplifying assumptions may be used temporarily when information is missing or is of poor quality, and permanently when removing relatively less important factors can make a model clearer or more useful.

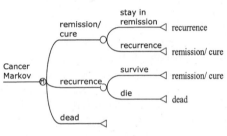

A Markov model

Monte Carlo simulation is used to deal with the related issues of variability and uncertainty in modeling. Distinctions are made in modeling between

- Variability across groups in a population, and
- Individual variability within groups,

and also between

- Error/uncertainty in estimating model parameters,
- Structural error/variability in models, and
- Stochastic uncertainty inherent in system events (e.g., rolls of dice).

Monte Carlo simulation of health economic models is of interest primarily as an advanced form of sensitivity analysis on uncertain parameters. The deterministic analysis of a model is repeated for a large number of sets of parameter values, as in a nonsimulation sensitivity analysis. In a simulation, however, values are drawn from realistic probability distributions randomly—thus "Monte Carlo"—and then statistical analysis is performed on the collected results. This is referred to as **probabilistic sensitivity analysis**.

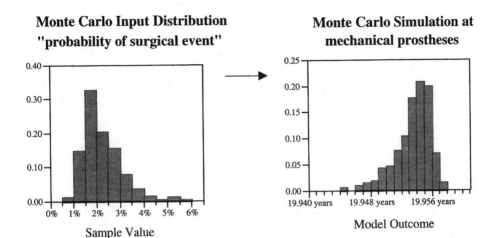

**Monte Carlo Input Distribution "probability of surgical event"**

Sample Value

**Monte Carlo Simulation at mechanical prostheses**

Model Outcome

Most analytical models include within their structure important stochastic uncertainties (i.e., an event whose outcome for a particular individual has a random element), the impact of which can be captured in the deterministic analysis of the model. Some complex models, particularly Markov models, can end up having too many stochastic uncertainties, which prevents their inclusion as part of the model's structure. In such cases, Monte Carlo simulation can be used to introduce the additional stochastic uncertainty into the operation of the model. Instead of a single deterministic calculation of the model, a large number of "individuals" are randomly walked through the uncertain events in the model, and statistical analysis is used on the aggregated results (simulation mean substituting for a deterministic value). This is referred to as **stochastic sensitivity analysis.**

During Monte Carlo simulation sensitivity analysis, the other forms of variability and uncertainty addressed by simulation (e.g., stochastic analysis) should be isolated from parameter uncertainty, using separate simulation "loops."

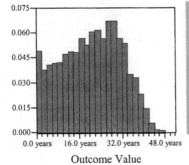

**Monte Carlo Simulation 3000 patients at mechanical prostheses**

Outcome Value

| Mean Value: | 20.0 years |
| Mode: | 27.0 years |
| Std Dev: | 11.0 years |
| Minimum Value: | 0.0 years |
| 2.5% | 0.0 years |
| Median: | 21.0 years |
| 97.5% | 39.0 years |
| Maximum Value: | 47.0 years |

## VALUE AND USE

By combining evidence from clinical trials with expert opinion and clinical experience, models and simulation can be used to explore the potential impacts of a decision or an intervention in clinical practice, before actually implementing the decision or intervention. As the term "health economics" suggests, the "impacts" being modeled can cover both health outcomes for patients and economic consequences for payers.

In addition to their use in internal decision making and in research publications, pharmacoeconomic models are increasingly a required part of submissions of evidence to external agencies, private and governmental, for use in formulary decision making.

Other aspects of modeling in pharmacoeconomics/health economics include

- Predicting long term outcomes from surrogate markers,
- Providing evidence-based estimates for data that have not been measured (e.g., base a model on one population and localize it to different populations),
- Extrapolating from existing data (e.g., base a hypothetical population model on evidence from a small number of cases),
- Analyzing many different subgroups, scenarios, and strategies, and
- Tailoring a population model to an individual.

In models such as decision trees that combine visual and analytical elements, the visual representation of the model can make it easier to construct the analytical model, and at the same time it improves the potential receptivity of an audience, so that reviewers of the model will be better able to

- Understand the analytical model,
- Understand and/or accept its results (particularly important in pharmacoeconomic models where the underlying data may be from diverse sources and of varying quality), and
- Make informed choices based on it.

Monte Carlo simulation is used primarily to assess the level of confidence in the results of a model (and in the recommendations of decision analyses and cost-effectiveness analyses derived from it). Monte Carlo simulation may also be used if the questions to be addressed by an analytical model include the distribution of potential outcomes ("risk analysis"). Relatively simple models can be subject to a deterministic risk analysis without simulation. However, if the model is a Markov model, then a deterministic analysis of the model will not be able to generate the distribution of likely outcomes. This is also true of models in which important parameters are assigned point values, while in reality they would be observed to be stochastic—having some kind of probability distribution. In such cases, a stochastic risk analysis can be performed using Monte Carlo simulation.

## ISSUES

Issues of nontransparency and perceived bias have to some extent slowed the acceptance of cost and effectiveness results and recommendations based on pharmacoeconomic models. Modelers can try to address such concerns by being transparent in their model structure and documenting justification and support for model inputs. Typically authors submitting manuscripts for publications based on models also submit detailed aspects of the model for consideration by the editor(s) and reviewers. Also to counter such negative perceptions, modelers will sometimes make model structure and/or input decisions that explicitly bias against the novel intervention. Clearly, all nontrivial model assumptions need to be clearly documented.

A related issue is the increasing use of more complex model forms, such as Markov processes, and the difficulties these pose for both internal and external validation. While having the potential for more accurate representation of natural histories of disease, the complex Markov models and accompanying Monte Carlo simulations found in research intended for publication may be opaque to reviewers—and, if published, remain mostly unavailable to expert, critical readers. Again, if modelers want their work to be accepted, it is in their interest to be as transparent as possible regarding their model structure and inputs.

Essentially all modeling guides focus heavily on the importance of thorough sensitivity analysis in proving the robustness of the model and the assumptions upon which it depends. There is typically misunderstanding about the different types of uncertainty and variability in models and how to handle them during analysis.

Health economics modeling and simulation is a relatively young discipline, and it is just beginning to benefit from easier availability of detailed modeling guidelines and tutorials. The ISPOR Good Research Practices Task Force report (Weinstein 2003) provides clear expectations for the kind of testing, calibration, and validation of models that should be done by the model builder before publishing model results. It also provides a detailed approach for assessing the quality of models.

BIBLIOGRAPHY

Gold MR, Siegel JE, Russell LB, Weinstein MC. *Cost-Effectiveness in Health and Medicine.* New York: Oxford University Press; 1996.

Hunink M, Glasziou P, Elstein A. *Decision Making in Health and Medicine.* Cambridge, UK: Cambridge University Press; 2001.

Weinstein MC, O'Brien B, Hornbberger J. Principles of good practice for decision analytic modeling in health-care evaluation. *Value Health.* 2003; 6:9–17.

# Monetary Value
## Constant Dollars
## Current Dollars

### BRIEF DEFINITION

Monetary value is a measure of the amount of currency that a buyer would be willing to exchange for a good, service, or resource, or the amount of currency that a seller would require to sell a good, service, or resource. Monetary value can be expressed as **constant dollars** or **current dollars**.

## EXPLANATION

"Value" is the amount of consumer satisfaction directly or indirectly obtained from a good, service, or resource. Different people value things differently according to personal taste, needs, and desires. Monetary value is a measure of the amount of money accepted by buyers and sellers as a sufficient amount in exchange for a good, service, or resource. Constant dollars are expressed in terms of their purchasing power in a base year. Constant dollars adjust for changes in buying power due to inflation or deflation between the base year and the year of measurement. Current dollars reflect the value of dollars spent or received at the time of the transaction, without adjusting for inflation or deflation since the transaction date.

## VALUE AND USE

Monetary value is similar to market value, which is the price at which a buyer is willing to buy and a seller is willing to sell. Constant dollars are also referred to as real dollars. When costs have been converted to constant dollars, the base year should be reported (e.g., 2001 US$). Current dollars are also referred to as nominal dollars.

## ISSUES

It is important to determine how monetary value is estimated. Considerations include the year and currency in which the good, service, or resource is valued and whether adjustments for inflation and deflation have been made (constant dollars) or not been made (current dollars). When comparing cost estimates reported in different years, it is necessary first to convert costs to constant dollars using an inflation adjustment factor.

## BIBLIOGRAPHY

Kumaranayake L. The real and the nominal? Making inflationary adjustments to cost and other economic data. *Health Policy Plan.* 2000;15:230–234.

# Monitoring Entity – Clinical Trials
**Institutional Review Board (IRB)**
**Data and Safety Monitoring Board (DSMB)**
**Independent Data Monitoring Committee**

## BRIEF DEFINITION

A **monitoring entity** is a group of individuals charged with ensuring compliance with rules and regulations. There are several levels of monitors that ensure compliance with regulations involving research on animals or humans in educational and research facilities, granting agencies, and research practice sites. Examples of such monitoring committees include **institutional review board (IRB)**, **data and safety monitoring board (DSMB)**, and **independent data monitoring committee** (*see term:* Research Entities).

## EXPLANATION

Monitoring boards in human or animal research have been developed to ensure compliance with ethical concerns raised in the Nuremberg Trials and the World Medical Association Declaration of Helsinki (I and II), which have been expanded on in the United States by the Code of Federal Regulations, Title 45, Part 46 "Protection of Human Subjects."

Institutions receiving federal support in the United States are required to have an IRB, which approves and oversees research involving human subjects. In addition, federal granting agencies require that grantees have in place procedures for insuring the safety of participants, validity of data, and termination of studies for which new and significant risks or benefits have been determined during the study, usually administered through the appropriate IRB. Granting agencies further reserve the right to conduct audits to ensure that all ethical and reporting requirements are met. Many other countries have similar committees. Although the basic principles governing their operation are similar, the specific rules and regulations regarding them may differ among countries.

The IRB is charged with assuring that studies have clearly defined endpoints and acceptable risk-to-benefit ratios. They must also ensure that informed consent is obtained from research subjects when appropriate and that the forms are understandable and free from coercive or misleading language. The IRB is also responsible for monitoring and reviewing the progress and changes to risks or benefits of a study.

The US National Institutes of Health further requires that funded clinical studies involving multiple sites have in place a DSMB, whose functions and oversight of safety and monitoring issues are distinct from the study review and approval provided by an IRB. These issues are typically specific to the research center and study, but include review of screening, baseline, efficacy, safety, and quality assurance data as well as other operational requirements. A DSMB allow for the collection and reporting of data from many sites that may not otherwise be shared and are not evaluated by an IRB.

## VALUE AND USE

Monitoring entities attempt to ensure ethical conduct in human and animal research. In addition, boards such as the IRB serve to define acceptable risk-to-benefit ratios when conducting research. The IRB protects both the researcher and the institution by assuring the community in which the research is being conducted that local ethical preferences have been considered. In the event of an adverse outcome, review of a research project by an IRB can provide some protection from litigation to both the researchers and the institution.

The monitoring requirements of a DSMB are much more rigid than those of an IRB and are recommended when large numbers of patients are involved or when the risks of a study are particularly high, such as in early human studies involving pharmaceuticals or in cancer therapies. Close surveillance of adverse events or lack of efficacy may result in early termination of a study, protecting human subjects from further harm.

ISSUES

Monitoring entities may vary considerably among countries and even regions. Acceptable research practice depends on a valuation of risk and benefit, which may vary considerably depending on culture. The degree to which monitoring boards require reporting of research is also highly variable and dependent upon its assessed risks and benefits. Reporting requirements continue to change over time and with changes in culture and technology.

BIBLIOGRAPHY

McFadden E. *Management of data in clinical trials.* New York: John Wiley & Sons, Inc; 1998.

National Institute on Drug Abuse. Data and safety monitoring board standard operating procedures. http://www.nida.nih.gov/Funding/DSMBSOP.html. Accessed March 31, 2003.

National Institutes of Health. NIH guide: NIH policy for data and safety monitoring. Released June 10, 1998. http://grants.nih.gov/grants/guide/notice-files/not98-084.html. Accessed March 31, 2003.

Redshaw ME, Harris A, Baum JD. Research ethics committee audit: differences between committees. *J Med Ethics.* 1996;22:78–82.

Swerdlow PS. Use of humans in biomedical experimentation. In: Macrina FL, ed. *Scientific integrity: an introductory text with cases.* Washington, DC: ASM Press; 1995.

# National Institute of Clinical Excellence (NICE)

BRIEF DEFINITION

The National Institute of Clinical Excellence (NICE) is a quasi-governmental organization that attempts to provide patients, health professionals, and the public in England and Wales with authoritative, robust, and reliable guidance on current medical "best practice."

EXPLANATION

NICE was created in April 1999 under the auspices of the National Health Service (NHS). The role of the institute encompasses the progression from evidence of clinical efficacy (used as the basis of decision making in the regulatory environment) toward clinical effectiveness and cost-effectiveness. This information is vital in the realm of actual clinical practice, and hence NICE has an extremely important role to play in health care decision making in England and Wales. NICE was formed to appraise medical technologies and devices. To date the majority of its work has related to medical technologies—that is, therapeutic interventions.

Explicitly NICE has declared that its role is to provide "guidance." NICE provides three types of guidance: "technology appraisals" of new and existing health technologies, "clinical guidelines" for the management of specific conditions, and "clinical audit methods" to support the technology appraisals and clinical guidelines. It is still expected that decisions will be made by the health care provider in light of this guidance based upon the needs of the patient. However, in reality the guidance is rarely ignored. The Commission for Health Improvement (CHI) has the responsibility for monitoring the acceptance of NICE guidances and to ensure that they are being followed. In cases where a guidance is being ignored, this must be justified in detail.

The NICE process (see figure) begins with a request from the Department of Health in England or the National Assembly for Wales to appraise a given technology. This request is typically based upon the likely impact of the technology upon the health status of patients and/or the financial impact for the NHS. At this time NICE invites all interested parties (companies, patient groups, etc) to submit their evidence. NICE also commissions an independent body to conduct an assessment of the technology. This information becomes a vital component of the overall appraisal. There are currently six centers across the United Kingdom that can undertake these assessments (Health Economics Centres at the Universities at York, Birmingham, Sheffield, Southampton, Aberdeenshire, and Liverpool).

The submission made by pharmaceutical/device companies is divided into five sections:

1. Disease background

2. Description of the technology

3. Clinical effectiveness

4. Cost effectiveness

5. Wider implications to the NHS

A revised guidance recently issued by the institute incorporates the rationale for each of these components of information.

NICE has access to privileged data in that companies may share information that is confidential in nature—for example, results from on-going trials and plans for extension of the current license. The information submitted is reviewed at a meeting of the appraisal committee. The committee brings together experts from the all the related areas—for example, consultants, health care providers, health economists, statisticians, and NHS executives. After this initial meeting, the appraisal committee releases to all involved parties the Provisional Appraisal Document (PAD)—or what is now called the Appraisal Consultation Document (ACD). A detailed description of the revised appraisal process and an updated synopsis of the process can be found in the new "Guide to the Technology Appraisal Process," accessible through the NICE Web site. The parties have a period of 28 days to provide a response to the PAD. After this period the appraisal committee meets again and this time issues the Final Appraisal Document (FAD). At this stage, the parties involved in the submissions have an opportunity to lodge any appeals, although the reasons for which appeals can be made are explicitly defined. Finally, the institute issues the final guidance through its Web site and through a publication.

VALUE AND USE

NICE is regarded globally as an important institution that assesses the value of new and existing therapies based upon an independent review by relevant experts. The effectiveness and progress of NICE is followed closely around the world.

ISSUES

One of the major issues surrounding NICE relates to its authority. As mentioned above, although NICE provides guidance, the clinical decision maker still makes the final decision based upon clinical judgment with respect to the needs of the individual patient. This implies that adherence with NICE guidance is not necessarily universal. Legal action to ensure compliance with the NICE guidance has been proposed.

A second important issue relates to the submissions by manufacturers. As mentioned earlier, NICE is in a privileged position insofar as it has access to unpublished data from manufacturers. Since the data is confidential—even if it provides key evidence for the appraisal—it cannot be disclosed in the guidance. The ability of those outside of NICE to evaluate the outcome may be limited in these cases. It has been suggested that NICE appraisals be made only when such

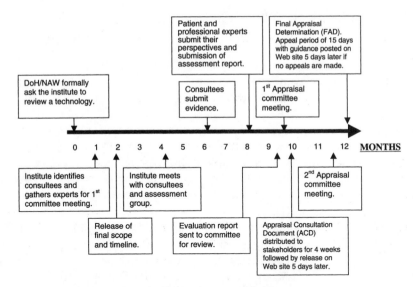

The NICE Technology Appraisal Process
Adapted from NICE Technology Appraisal Process. www.nice.org.uk

key information is in the public domain—that is, at the time of launch or two to three years postlaunch. The resolution of this issue will clearly have a significant impact on the ultimate influence of NICE guidance.

BIBLIOGRAPHY

Littlejohns P. The national institute for clinical excellence: Its importance and implications for the pharmaceutical industry. *Drug Inf J.* 2001;35:181–188.

NICE. www.nice.org.uk. Accessed March 31, 2003.

Rawlins M. In pursuit of quality: The national institute of clinical excellence. Lancet. 1999; 353:1079–1082.

# Net Benefit
## Net Monetary Benefit
## Net Health Benefit
## Incremental Net Benefit

### BRIEF DEFINITION

**Net benefit** is an alternative method of displaying cost-effectiveness results (alternative to the cost-effectiveness ratio) (*see terms:* Cost-Benefit Analysis, Cost-Effectiveness Acceptability Curve, Cost-Effectiveness Analysis, Cost-Utility Analysis). When it is expressed in monetary units it is formally a **net monetary benefit**, whereas when expressed in units of efficacy or utility it is called a **net health benefit**. When two treatments are compared, the difference between the two should be referred to as an **incremental net benefit**.

## EXPLANATION

Let the difference in mean costs between Treatment 2 and Treatment 1 be denoted by $\Delta_c = C_2 - C_1$ and let the difference in mean efficacy (or effectiveness) between Treatment 2 and Treatment 1 be $\Delta_E = E_2 - E_1$. Then the familiar incremental cost-effectiveness ratio (ICER) (*see term:* Cost-Effectiveness Analysis) for Treatment 2 against Treatment 1 is $\Delta_c/\Delta_E$. The ICER is traditionally, although not universally, compared with a threshold willingness-to-pay K (e.g., \$50 000/quality-adjusted life year gained), such that if the ICER is less than K, then Treatment 2 should be accepted as cost-effective relative to Treatment 1.

The cost-effectiveness plane was introduced by Black (1990) and is shown

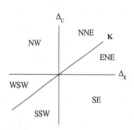

The cost-effectiveness plane

in the figure. The true value of the efficacy and cost differences between treatments is expressed as a point $(\Delta_E, \Delta_c)$ on this plane. In the area above the axis marked $\Delta_E$ the cost difference is positive, while in that to the right of the axis marked $\Delta_c$ the efficacy difference is positive. The southeast quadrant, labeled "SE," therefore has positive efficacy difference but negative cost difference, and so, if the true point lies in this quadrant, Treatment 2 dominates Treatment 1. Generally, if one wishes to demonstrate cost-effectiveness of Treatment 2, it is preferable to be as far to the south and east as possible. Conversely, in the "NW" quadrant, Treatment 1 dominates. A line of slope K divides the northeast and southwest quadrants. A point in the sector marked "ENE" represents a case in which Treatment 2 is more effective than Treatment 1 but is also more costly. Neither treatment dominates, but the efficacy difference is sufficiently large relative to the cost difference for Treatment 2 to be preferable to Treatment 1. Similarly, a point in the "SSW" sector represents the case where Treatment 2 is less effective than Treatment 1 but is less costly, and the cost difference is sufficiently large relative to the efficacy difference for Treatment 2 to be more cost-effective.

Generally, then, Treatment 2 is more cost-effective than Treatment 1 for all points below the line of slope K. In contrast, the ICER is less than K for all points in the regions labeled "ENE," "SE," "WSW," and "NW" in the figure. Notice that this actually includes the northwest quadrant in which Treatment 1 dominates. This is why cost-effectiveness comparison is not just a question of whether the ICER is less than *K*. It is also necessary to consider the sign of $\Delta_E$. If this is negative, then we prefer Treatment 2 only if the ICER is *greater* than *K*. Traditionally in cost-effectiveness analysis this is handled by using a two-step approach. First, one checks for dominance (*see term:* Dominance): that is, is the point in the SE or NW quadrants? If there is dominance, the decision is made on that basis. If there is not dominance, the ICER is used. This is another reason why working with the ICER is unnecessarily complex. After all, what we really wish to know is very simple: does the point $(\Delta_E, \Delta_C)$ lie below the sloping line?

Several authors who have advocated an approach based on net benefits have made this argument. The net monetary benefit of Treatment 2 against Treatment 1 is defined to be $K \Delta_E - \Delta_C$, while the net health benefit is $\Delta_E - \Delta_C/K$. They differ only in that the net monetary benefit is expressed in units of money while the net health benefit is expressed in units of efficacy. Both have the property that they are positive if, and only if, the point $(\Delta_E, \Delta_C)$ lies below the sloping line in the cost-effectiveness plane.

Because it is a linear function of $\Delta_E$ and $\Delta_C$, statistical inference about net benefit is considerably more straightforward than inference about the ICER.

## VALUE AND USE

It should be noted that, although usually defined as above in terms of cost-effectiveness, the net benefit approach is equally valid and valuable in contexts usually called cost-utility or cost-benefit analysis in health economics. We have referred to $\Delta_E$ as the mean difference in efficacy, but it could equally well be in units of utility—for example, quality-adjusted life years—or some other measure of benefit.

Since the definition of net benefits is dependent on the threshold willingness-to-pay K, the usual way to present a cost-effectiveness analysis using net benefits is through a cost-effectiveness acceptability curve (CEAC). The CEAC plots the probability that net benefit is positive as a function of K. Note that this probability is the same for a given K, whether we are working in terms of net health benefit or net monetary benefit.

## ISSUES

Although the net benefit approach is gaining adherents in health economics, the ICER is still the dominant approach to assessing cost-effectiveness. As a single point estimate of cost-effectiveness, an estimate of the ICER is arguably the most useful, although it is important to also know the sign of $\Delta_E$, or equivalently to use the two-step approach of first checking for dominance. However, it is invariably important to quantify uncertainty about cost-effectiveness. A confidence interval for the ICER is more complex to construct and to interpret because of the way the ratio switches sign as the sign of $\Delta_E$ changes. The simplicity of the net benefit approach is then attractive, and the CEAC provides a cost-effectiveness summary that is of direct relevance to decision makers.

## BIBLIOGRAPHY

Black WC. The CE plane: a graphic representation of cost-effectiveness. *Med Decis Making.* 1990;10:212–214.

Stinnett AA, Mulahy J. Net health benefits: A new framework for the analysis of uncertainty in cost-effectiveness analysis. *Medical Decis Making.* 1998;18(suppl):S68–S80.

# New Drug Application (NDA)

Investigational New Drug Application (IND)
Abbreviated New Drug Application (ANDA)
Supplemental New Drug Application (SNDA)
Approvable Letter
Approval Letter
Not Approvable Letter

### BRIEF DEFINITION

A **New Drug Application** (NDA) is the documentation provided as evidence supporting the safety and effectiveness of a new pharmaceutical in order to obtain approval by the US Food and Drug Administration (FDA) (*see term:* Food and Drug Administration) for its commercial marketing.

### EXPLANATION

The NDA process, established in 1938, requires all new drugs in the United States to be reviewed and approved prior to sale and marketing. The FDA is an agency of the federal government within the Department of Health and Human Services. Within the FDA, the Center for Drug Evaluation and Research (CDER) is responsible for review of NDAs.

Before a sponsor company can submit an NDA, it must first file an acceptable **Investigational New Drug Application** (IND) to begin clinical studies. The data collected under the IND is combined with other data on the drug and its manufacture to complete the documentation required for a complete NDA.

The FDA reviewer of an NDA should have enough information to be able verify that the drug is safe and effective for its proposed use(s) and that the drug benefits outweigh the potential risks. Also, the NDA should demonstrate appropriate labeling and describe the manufacturing methods used to make the product. Other information that should be found in the NDA include: drug ingredients; the condition and patients to be treated; the appropriate dose(s) and duration(s) of therapy; all signs, symptoms, and responses measured; and side effects and adverse effects. Specific information and the application for FDA approval to market a new drug can be found in section 21 of the Code of Federal Regulations (CFR), part 314. This section of the CFR is the FDA interpretation of the Federal Food, Drug, and Cosmetic Act and related statutes.

An **Abbreviated New Drug Application** (ANDA) requires less information than an NDA and is submitted by a sponsor company when it wishes to gain approval to market a generic drug. A **Supplemental New Drug Application** (SNDA) may be submitted for consideration of a new indication for a previously approved drug.

Once the FDA has received an NDA submission, the agency will determine within 60 days whether the application may be filed. This is a prereview time to decide whether the application contains adequate information to proceed with the in-depth review. If the NDA is filed, the 180-day in-depth review process, otherwise known as the "review clock," will begin on the filing date. During the "review clock" the FDA will make a decision to issue an approvable, approval, or not approvable letter. An **approvable letter** is a written statement by the FDA stating the NDA will be accepted when additional information is submitted or under other specific conditions. The **approval letter** is a written statement by the FDA stating that the NDA has been accepted. The **not approvable letter** is a written statement by the FDA stating that the NDA has not been approved.

### VALUE AND USE

To sell and market a new drug entity in the United States, an NDA must be approved as required by federal law. Any actions that fall outside the regulations are punishable in a court of law.

### ISSUES

Understanding the process and rationale that CDER uses for evaluating an NDA can be important and can help the progression toward gaining an approval letter. CDER offers assistance at various times during the application process through scheduled meetings or guidance documents. The guidance documents are not enforceable as regulation or law but are useful to follow because they represent the current thinking of CDER on specific subjects and can save time in the review process for the sponsor company.

### BIBLIOGRAPHY

Clair AG, Millstein LG. General Considerations of the NDA. In: Guarino RA, ed. *New Drug Approval Process.* 2nd ed. New York: Marcel Dekker, Inc; 1993.

CFR §314 revised, p. 101–103. April 1, 1998. Available at http://www.access.gpo.gov/nara/cfr/waisidx_98/21cfr314_98.html. Accessed March 31, 2003.

United States Food and Drug Administration, Center for Drug Evaluation and Research. Drug Applications. http://www.fda.gov/cder/regulatory/applications/nda.htm. Accessed February 8, 2002.

# Number Needed to Treat (NNT)

### BRIEF DEFINITION

**Number needed to treat** (NNT) means the average number of patients needed to be treated for a specific period of time to observe one less adverse event by the end of the period.

### EXPLANATION

Introduced by Laupacis in 1988 (Laupacis et al, 1988), the term "number-needed-to-treat" has gained widespread use in the medical community and medical journals. A graphic representation may ease the understanding of NNT. Figure 1 depicts a hypothetical randomized trial aimed at treating a fatal disease in 20 pairs of patients. In each pair of identical patients, one receives

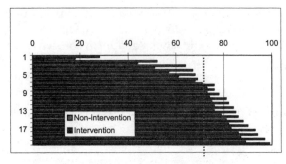

Figure 1. Survival times in a hypothetical trial in which
pairs of identical patients have either intervention or
nonintervention. Survival time is shown on the
X-axis and patient number on the Y-axis.

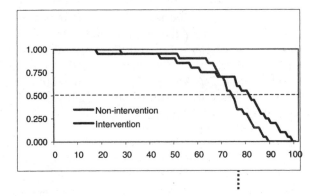

Figure 2. The same trial depicted with survival curves.
Survival time is shown on the X-axis and proportion alive on
the Y-axis. $M_i$ and $M_c$ are the proportions with fatal outcome
in the intervention group and control groups. The distance
between the two survival curves along the horizontal dotted
line indicates the gain in median survival time.

active therapy while the other receives placebo. Because each pair is identical, the effect of the therapy can be observed directly by measuring survival time in the patient receiving active therapy and in the control patient.

Early during the trial, patients on therapy fare worse than the controls, while later in the trial patients on therapy benefit (Figure 1). Usually, the results of a trial are shown with the proportion surviving on the Y-axis as in Figure 2. The effect of the therapy can now be expressed with different types of measures. The vertical measures capture effects at an arbitrary point in time (for example the vertical dotted line). If at this point in time, $M_c$ and $M_i$ are the proportions with fatal outcome in the control group and intervention group respectively, the effects can be expressed in the following way:

(1) Relative risk reduction (RRR): $(M_c - M_i)/M_i$
(2) Absolute risk reduction (ARR): $M_c - M_i$
The reciprocal of ARR is NNT:
(3) Number-needed-to-treat (NNT): $1/ARR$

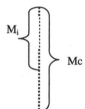

$M_c$ and $M_i$ can also be formulated as odds ratio and log odds ratio.
All five vertical measures are different mathematical formulations of the two proportions $M_c$ and $M_i$. None of these five measures are more correct than the others; they simply express different aspects of the intervention effect.

## VALUE AND USE

It has become customary to define NNT as "the number of patients needed to be treated for $x$ years to avoid one bad outcome." This definition, however, is not correct. First, NNT represents an *average* number. Second, adverse outcomes are not avoided altogether, they are just postponed, as can be seen in Figure 1.

The use of NNT has been expanded to encompass harm "("number needed to harm," or NNH), screening ("number needed to screen"), education ("number needed to educate"), and exposure ("number needed to expose").

NNT does not inform about the proportion of patients that benefit positively or negatively from an intervention. In Figure 1, NNT is 20 at the vertical dotted line, and still all patients having therapy are influenced, positively or negatively, by it. From a biological point of view, it is plausible that interventions have a small effect in many patients rather than a large effect in a few.

The confidence limits of NNT are usually taken as the reciprocal of the confidence limits of ARR even though this method may create a biased confidence interval (Hutton 2000). When the confidence interval of ARR contains zero (for example $[-0.02, +0.05]$), NNT has two confidence intervals (in the example: $[-\infty, -50]$ and $[+20, +\infty]$). The confidence interval of NNT is undefined in the interval $[-1, +1]$ because one needs to treat at least one patient to avoid or induce an adverse outcome.

## ISSUES

Because ARR can vary considerably in time, NNT will also vary. Therefore, NNT may for example be 50 after 1 year of therapy, 75 after 2 years and 40 after 3 years. Also, NNT varies with the baseline risk of adverse events in the control group. Consequently, NNT is not a number that is specific for a therapy or a group of patients.

Figure 2 illustrates two other types of effect measures. The horizontal effect measures capture the horizontal difference between the two survival curves. Gain in median survival time is a measure frequently used in cancer research. Gain in life expectancy is a combined effect measure that captures survival time as well as survival probability. It is represented by the net area between the survival curves (Figure 2).

In Figures 1 and 2, the adverse event is death. The arguments would be the same if it were a nonfatal event such as myocardial infarction (MI). In that case the combined effect measure will express the expected gain in MI free survival. While fatal outcomes can be postponed but not prevented, nonfatal outcomes can be prevented in the sense that an intervention postpones the event to the extent that patients die from other causes.

There is ample evidence that patients, physicians, and health administrators are more likely to opt for an intervention when its effect is presented in terms of RRR than as ARR or NNT. Since there is no gold standard, it is unclear which measure is best. There is evidence that lay people (Kristiansen 2002) as well as physicians misunderstand NNT (Kristiansen 2003) and there is no evidence that NNT helps people make better decisions. Vertical effect measures might well be supplemented with combined measures in order to improve understanding among lay people and physicians. The use of NNT in economic evaluation may create misleading results and may be better avoided (Laupacis 1988). Economic evaluation should be based on life expectancy, not NNT.

BIBLIOGRAPHY

Halvorsen PA, Kristiansen IS, Aasland OG, Førde OH. Medical doctors' perception of the "number needed to treat" (NNT). A survey of Norwegian doctors' recommendations for two therapies with different NNT. *Scand J Prim Health Care.* 2003;21.

Hutton JL. Number needed to treat: properties and problems. *J R Stat Soc.* 2000;163:403–419.

Kristiansen IS, Gyrd-Hansen D. Cost-effectiveness analysis based on the number-needed-to-treat: common sense or non-sense? *Health Econ.* 2003;12: in press.

Kristiansen IS, Gyrd-Hansen D, Nexoe J, Nielsen JB. Number needed to treat: easily understood and intuitively meaningful? Theoretical considerations and a randomized trial. *J Clin Epidemiol.* 2002;55:888–892.

Laupacis A, Sackett DL, Roberts RS. An assessment of clinically useful measures of the consequences of treatment. *N Engl J Med.* 1988;318:1728–1733.

# Observational Study

## BRIEF DEFINITION

An **observational study** is a prospective research method for documenting clinical, economic, and/or humanistic outcomes of actual medical practice absent the constraints of a more formal experimental design (*see term:* Clinical Trial).

## EXPLANATION

To prove or disprove a hypothesis, a research study must be constructed so as to minimize extraneous variables that might impact upon the study's conclusion. Controlled clinical research is typified by statistical power, rigorous inclusion criteria, randomization, a rigid protocol, and predetermined measures and assessments. In most cases, the conditions that improve the statistical validity and overall credibility associated with findings from controlled clinical research differ considerably from those found in actual medical practice. Hence, the outcomes achieved in clinical research may not be representative of nor achievable in the "real world."

An observational study is undertaken to explore processes employed and outcomes achieved in settings more reflective of actual medical practice. In these studies, conducted prospectively, care must be taken to engineer benign approaches to data collection so as not to impact upon the conditions being observed. Even greater care must be placed on the interpretation of findings from observational studies, inasmuch as there is no guarantee of comparability between cohorts within the study. Propensity analysis and other advanced statistical techniques, however, can be employed to minimize the impact of confounding variables. While not considered to be as definitive as findings from controlled clinical trials, data from observational studies can prove to be a rich foundation upon which to explore relationships between outcomes and clinical processes, treatments, and disease characteristics.

## VALUE AND USE

A prospective observational study can represent an ideal platform for exploring the outcomes of medical care unencumbered by the often-artificial "protocol driven" components of controlled clinical research. As such, observational research can provide a reasonable basis for considering relative cost-effectiveness, for assessing quality of life, and for examining the frequency of reportable adverse events. Observational studies have been established in the form of patient registries to examine the link between use of a particular product and the occurrence of serious adverse events. In addition, patient registries have been established to examine directly the role of various therapies and treatment regimens in the management of specific diseases and conditions.

## ISSUES

Rarely is a prospective observational study based on a specific hypothesis. As such, they differ importantly and intrinsically from statistically powered controlled clinical trials. Rather than seeking to answer a specific question, however, an observational study is designed to be exploratory, or hypothesis generating. Nonetheless, important trends and statistically valid conclusions can be derived from observational study, provided that data collected are accurate and that advanced statistical techniques have been used to minimize confounding variables. The primary advantage of observational research is in its descriptions of actual medical practice, the actual patient population, and the impact of actual medical practice on the actual typical heterogeneous, patient population. Policymakers, regulatory agencies, drug and device companies, physicians, and patients are increasingly looking to observational research to better understand "what works" under "real-world" conditions.

## BIBLIOGRAPHY

Horwitz RI, Viscoli CM, Clemens JD, Sadock RT. Developing improved observational methods for evaluating therapeutic effectiveness. *Am J Med.* 1990;89:630–638.

Michels KB, Braunwald E. Estimating treatment effects from observational data. Dissonant and resonant notes from the SYMPHONY trials. *JAMA.* 2002;287:3130–3132.

Radford MJ, Foody JM. How do observational studies expand the evidence basis for therapy? *JAMA.* 2001;286:1149–1152.

Rosenbaum PR, Rubin DB. The central role of the propensity score in observational studies for causal effects. 1993;70:41–55.

# Outcomes Research

ECHO Model
Consequences
Clinical Intermediary
Clinical Outcomes
Humanistic Intermediary

Humanistic Outcomes
Costs
Economic Outcomes
Treatment Modifiers

## BRIEF DEFINITION

**Outcomes research** is the scientific discipline that evaluates the effect of health care interventions on patient-related, if not patient-specific, clinical, humanistic, and economic outcomes. Outcomes research is generally based on the conceptual framework that evaluation of treatment alternatives involves the simultaneous assessment of multiple types of outcomes that are disease-related.

## Explanation

A diagram of outcomes research–the ECHO model (economic, clinical, and humanistic outcomes) is shown below. Outcomes research–the ECHO model includes the following terminology.

**Consequences**: A general term used to refer to any effect related to the alternatives modeled (*see term:* Cost-Consequence Analysis).

**Clinical intermediary**: Measurements of a patient's physical or biomedical status used as a surrogate for or to infer the degree of disease (e.g., blood pressure, forced expiratory volume).

**Clinical outcomes**: Medical events that occur as a result of disease or treatment (e.g., stroke, disability, hospitalization) (*see terms:* Clinical Trial, Epidemiology, Pharmacoepidemiology).

**Humanistic intermediary**: Factors that affect the formation of patients' opinions about the effects of disease or treatment on their lives and well-being (e.g., values, norms, perceptions) (*see terms:* Health-Related Quality of Life, Patient-Reported Outcomes).

**Humanistic outcomes**: Patient self-assessment of the impact of disease or treatment on their lives and well-being (e.g., satisfaction, quality of life) (*see terms:* Health-Related Quality of Life, Patient-Reported Outcomes).

**Costs**: Direct medical, direct nonmedical, and indirect costs associated with the treatment alternatives evaluated (*see term:* Cost – Health Economics).

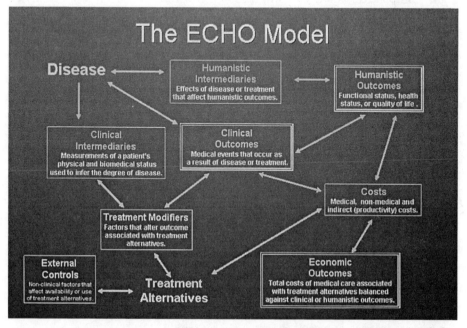

Figure reprinted from CM Kozma, CE Reeder, RM Schulz. Economic, clinical, and humanistic outcomes: A planning model for pharmacoeconomic research. *Clin Ther.* 1993;15:1121–32.

**Economic outcomes:** Direct and indirect costs compared to consequences of medical treatment alternatives typically expressed as ratios of cost to consequence (e.g., cost minimization, cost-effectiveness, cost utility, and cost-benefit ratios) (*see terms:* Cost-Benefit Analysis, Cost-Effectiveness Analysis, Cost-Minimization Analysis, Cost-Utility Analysis).

**Treatment modifiers:** Factors that may alter intermediaries or outcomes associated with treatment alternatives (e.g., side effects, compliance) (*see term:* Compliance).

In outcomes research, there is a distinction between outcomes (i.e., end results) and intermediaries (e.g., surrogate endpoints). It is an important distinction because it forces reflection on differences between "end results" and intermediaries. For example, blood pressure is a clinical intermediary in the treatment of hypertension while stroke or myocardial infarctions are clinical outcomes (i.e., end results). Distinction between intermediaries and outcomes is also important because it has implications for measurement such as reliability, validity, and duration of a study. While most researchers believe that there is a strong relationship between blood pressure and stroke, intermediaries for other diseases might not be as well established. The timing of data collection and size of sample required is also affected by choice of outcome or endpoint. Studying stroke rates requires much longer periods of time and much larger samples than does measuring blood pressure. The distinction between outcomes and intermediaries may also vary depending on the perspective taken for the analysis. For example, if a pharmacist is implementing a counseling program, compliance would be viewed as an "end result" from the pharmacist's perspective. However, from the perspective of a health care organization studying stroke, compliance may be viewed as an intermediary while the outcome of interest is survival.

When planning outcomes research, a societal perspective should be used for identification of consequences, even if this perspective is later restricted for a particular application. During the outcomes research planning process, specification of the disease or condition and selection of relevant alternatives for comparison is important. All consequences related to the treatment alternatives should then be listed for the patient populations of interest.

## VALUE AND USE

The outcomes research ECHO model represents only one of many available outcomes research models. The outcomes research ECHO model has been used extensively for teaching medical professionals about designing and reviewing outcomes research studies. The value is in using it prior to development of a study or evaluation of a body of literature. A priori specification of the factors that are important to the evaluator can lead to better decision making.

## BIBLIOGRAPHY

CM Kozma, CE Reeder, RM Schulz. Economic, clinical, and humanistic outcomes: A planning model for pharmacoeconomic research. *Clin Ther.* 1993;15:1121–1132.

# Patient-Reported Outcomes (PRO)

### BRIEF DEFINITION

**Patient-reported outcomes (PRO)** is an umbrella term that includes outcome data reported directly by the patient. It is one source of data that may be used to describe a patient's condition and response to treatment. It includes such outcomes as global impressions, functional status, well-being, symptoms, health-related quality of life (HRQL), satisfaction with treatment, and treatment adherence (*see terms:* Compliance, Health-Related Quality of Life).

### EXPLANATION

PRO is a term that has recently come into use. It was first proposed February 2001 at a meeting of the PRO Harmonization Group (a working group composed of members of the International Society for Pharmacoeconomics and Outcomes Research (ISPOR), International Society for Quality of Life Research (ISOQOL), the Pharmaceutical Research and Manufacturers of America Health Outcomes Committee (PhRMA-HOC), and the European Regulatory Issues on Quality of Life Assessment (ERIQA). While there has been a large increase in interest in understanding the patient's perspective of disease and treatment, the lack of a clear framework and agreed-upon terminology often has resulted in communication difficulties among researchers and with regulatory authorities. One approach to conceptualizing data collected in clinical trials is to consider the source of the data. There are several potential sources of data to evaluate the safety and efficacy of a new drug:

- Patient-reported outcomes (e.g., global impression, functional status, HRQL, symptoms)
- Caregiver-reported outcomes (e.g., dependency, functional status)
- Clinician-reported outcomes (e.g., global impressions, observations, tests of function)
- Physiological outcomes (e.g., FEV1, HbA1c, tumor size)

Each source serves as an umbrella term for the different types of data that may be provided by each source. The different sources have been shown to provide unique information regarding the efficacy of a therapy (e.g., Surarez-Almazor 2001; Rothman et al. 1991). The PRO component of the framework is based on the following assumptions:

- The patient's subjective experience provides a unique and valuable contribution to the drug development process.

- The information provided by the patient is inherently subjective.
- Scientific methods for assessing subjective outcomes (e.g., psychometrics and utility measurement) are well developed and provide the basis for PRO assessment.
- The design of PRO studies should follow the rules defined for other types of clinical trials (e.g., clear specification of hypotheses, standard methods of analysis and interpretation).

VALUE AND USE

The proposed framework recognizes the unique value of data from each source including patients. The appropriateness of using data from each source is context specific; that is, in some cases a PRO may be the best or only source of data while in other cases clinician-reported or multiple sources of outcome data may be most appropriate. This framework also encourages researchers to specify the type of PRO being assessed (e.g., symptoms, HRQL, functional status). This specificity is expected to facilitate communication among researchers and regulatory authorities.

ISSUES

This framework for clarifying patient outcomes assessment is proposed for use within the context of the drug development and regulatory process. Appropriateness of use beyond this context must be evaluated separately. It is recognized that PRO assessment is an evolving field; thus the proposed framework is intended to foster further research and enhance communication rather than be prescriptive.

BIBLIOGRAPHY

Acquadro C, Berzon R, Dubois D, et al. Incorporating the patient's perspective into drug development and communication: An ad hoc task force report of the Patient-Reported Outcomes (PRO) Harmonization Group meeting of the Food and Drug Administration, February 16, 2001. *Value Health.* 2003;6:522–531.

Rothman ML, Hedrick SC, Bulcroft KA, et al. The validity of proxy-generated scores as measures of patient health status. *Med Care.* 1991;29:115–124.

Surarez-Almazor ME, Conner-Spady B, Kendall CJ, et al. Lack of congruence in the ratings of patients' health status by patients and their physicians. *Med Decis Making.* 2001;21:113–121.

# Patient Rights

BRIEF DEFINITION

**Patient rights** refers to a complex set of principles of health care practice either specified by law or by the ethical doctrines of medical organizations and/or consumer groups aimed at protecting those who seek and/or obtain health care services; it also refers to the rights of patients who participate in clinical trials. These principles and ethical doctrines may vary depending upon whether the patient is a minor or an adult, is mentally competent to make decisions, or is incarcerated, or whether there is an immediate life threatening situation; they also may vary according to locality depending upon applicable local laws and regulations.

## EXPLANATION

In the United States, a federal Patient Bill of Rights has been subject to debate and proposed legislation in Congress. The basic legal rights of patients in the United States include being able to decide whether to accept or reject medical care, even life-saving care. Basic rights also include the ability to obtain one's own medical records, the right to refuse to participate in educational or research programs, and the right not to be discriminated against on the basis of race, color, national origin, gender, sexual orientation, or disability. Privacy protections are also included in certain federal, state, and local laws. Doctors have an obligation to provide information needed for patients to make decisions about medical care. Some documents on patient rights also include statements on patient responsibilities. Consumer groups and advocacy groups work on raising awareness about issues related to patient rights.

Various procedures and policy statements have been issued by medical organizations to protect patients participating in research programs. These include the World Medical Association Declaration of Helsinki that establishes ethical principles for medical research involving human subjects. Experimental research typically involves review of the protocol by an independent committee such as an Institutional Review Board. In addition, patients need to consent to participate in the research after having been supplied information on the potential benefits and risks of participation as well as information on sources of funding and potential conflicts of interest.

## VALUE AND USE

Goals of improved protection of patient rights and knowledge of patient responsibility include

- Improving consumer confidence by assuring that the health care system is fair and responsive to consumer needs and provides a mechanism for consumers to address their concerns,
- Supporting a strong relationship between patients and their health care providers, and
- Establishing rights and responsibilities of all participants (patients and providers) in improving patient health.

In addition, policy statements and laws on patient rights can provide guidance on the conduct of medical research and the delivery of medical services. Ultimately, the patient rights movement can improve the health and welfare of patients through improved research and health care delivery practices.

## ISSUES

The policies and laws that protect patient rights are evolving and complex. Some laws are tied to the operations of health plans and reimbursement policies of Medicare, Medicaid, or private insurers. Other rights are overseen by organizations that conduct research involving human subjects. There are laws including COBRA (Consolidated Omnibus Reconciliation Act) that provide certain rights when the participation in health benefits may be interrupted by unemployment, divorce, or death in the family. Additional protection related to privacy of medical information and protection on insurability when health insurance is discontinued due to certain life events is part of HIPAA (the Health Insurance Portability and Accountability Act) legislation. Some of these policies may be administered through the benefits programs offered by employers. The Department of Labor also has policies to protect the health and welfare of employees. An internet search on the term "Patient Rights" resulted in over 2,910,000 entries. Many of these sites were developed by individual health care organizations and contained postings of the organization's policy on patient rights. Additional rights that some of these organizations aim for included the expectation for prompt and courteous service, the right to ask questions, and timely results from tests and procedures. There are many organizations and professional groups involved in work related to the protection of patient rights.

BIBLIOGRAPHY

Declaration of Helsinki. www.wma.net. Accessed March 31, 2003.
National Coalition for Patient Rights. www.health.gov/nhic/NHICScripts/Entry.cfm?HRCode= HR3345. Accessed March 31, 2003.
Office of Human Subject Research Protection. ohrp.osophs.dhhs.gov. Accessed March 31, 2003.
Patient Rights and Responsibilities, The Quality Interagency Coordination Task Force (QuIC). www.consumer.gov/qualityhealth/rights.htm. Accessed March 31, 2003.
Patient Rights at Your Fingertips, Patient Rights Program, Boston University School of Public Health, Health Law Department. www.patient-rights.org. Accessed March 31, 2003.

# Patient Study Recruitment

BRIEF DEFINITION

**Patient study recruitment** is the process of enrolling patients and other volunteers into a clinical research study, such as a clinical trial. The total process spans several stages, from identifying the types of study participants desired to obtaining informed consent from protocol eligible individuals who have satisfied study admission criteria.

EXPLANATION

Establishing the patient study recruitment plan early in a research study is important. The protocol design and requirements identify the types of study participants desired, thus establishing the study admission criteria. The study research staff must explore the various sources that may yield potentially eligible study candidates. One obvious source is an investigator's own medical practice. Another source is the referral by another physician, suggesting that an individual be considered for a particular study. Some studies seek to enroll patients who have a particular diagnosis or specific characteristics in their medical history. Medical records, patient registries, and clinical databases can be good sources of such information, but special precautions to respect patient privacy must be considered and implemented if these are to be used as a source for potential study participants. If the medical condition or problem to be researched in the study is fairly common, self-referrals may be adequate. A patient is considered a self-refer if he or she responded to external recruitment efforts such as advertising. Another source of potential participants is mass screening in a community. This process highlights a specific disease or condition, offers screening to the general population, and offers referral information and information about a specific research study to those who may be qualified to enroll. Mass screenings can be conducted at health fairs, shopping malls, drugstores, or even in mobile vans that are equipped for testing.

Whatever the source used to identify potential study participants, a good screening plan is essential to the success of the study. During the initial screening, the study team must assess the study candidate's interest by describing the amount of effort and the risks involved in the study. The candidate must meet all study admission criteria; that is, he or she must possess all the characteristics in the inclusion criteria and have none of those identified in the exclusion criteria. Some studies may require that clinical tests be performed during the screening of a study candidate, the results of which are to be used in determining eligibility. If the patient is eligible and wishes to volunteer for the study, the investigator must obtain the patient's informed consent prior to the start of any study procedures. Informed consent refers to a person's voluntary agreement (free of coercion) to participate in research, based on adequate knowledge and understanding of relevant information. It should be noted that if screening tests are performed solely for study eligibility and would not have been performed otherwise, then patient informed consent must be obtained prior to the conduct of the screening tests.

## VALUE AND USE

Slow patient enrollment is the primary reason for delay in clinical studies. As a result, timely enrollment of patients into studies is of paramount importance to sponsoring organizations. Failure to recruit the necessary number of participants within a specific time frame may prevent the successful completion of a study within the originally anticipated budget. Sponsoring organizations view patient study recruiting in terms of enrollment and retention. An argument can be made that the patient recruitment process directly impacts patient retention. The human interaction that begins with the methods used by sites to reach potential study participants is a critical link to patient retention. The methods should be simple, direct, truthful, and noncoercive. Such methods include forms of advertising such as the use of posters and flyers and the use of media such as radio, television, newspapers, magazines, and journals. Advertising campaigns are especially important since two-thirds of enrolling patients into studies are by a self-referral. A new trend in patient recruiting is the use of Web sites on the Internet. There are roughly 83 million people in the United States using the Internet at home. Many of these people are specifically searching for health-related information. Many clinical research sites, government agencies, and professional recruiting groups have created Web sites that identify clinical studies and provide contact information.

ISSUES

As sponsoring organizations outsource more study activities, investigative research sites will assume more responsibility for patient study enrollment. It is critical that site investigators plan early for recruitment strategies and factor this study component into the study budget. Special attention and consideration should be given to the resources needed to carry out the recruitment plan. This includes staff to initiate the recruiting efforts as well as staff to handle the results of the recruiting efforts. In today's competitive market, sponsoring organizations usually understand the need for funds to support patient recruitment activities.

Not only is the research study team concerned with the safety and well-being of the study participants; it must also be concerned with patient privacy and confidentiality issues. Under federal regulations, the local institutional review board (IRB) must review and approve all methods used to recruit people into any research study. The IRB must ensure that the methods are not coercive and that the confidentiality and privacy of potential research participants are protected. When a potential study candidate is identified through medical records, databases, registries, or physician referrals, the primary physician must give approval for his or her patient to be contacted for research purposes. The patient's primary physician or caregiver should do any initial contact based upon private and identifiable medical information. In addition, the IRB must review and approve the text of all advertisements. Failure to include this material in the study application to the IRB could result in further delays in patient enrollment.

BIBLIOGRAPHY

Anderson D. *A Guide to Patient Recruitment.* Boston: CenterWatch, Inc; 2001.
Spilker B, Cramer JA. *Patient Recruitment in Clinical Trials.* New York: Raven Press; 1992.

# Pharmacoeconomics

BRIEF DEFINITION

**Pharmacoeconomics** is the scientific discipline that assesses the overall value of pharmaceutical health care products, services, and programs. Of necessity, it addresses the clinical, economic, and humanistic aspects of health care interventions in the prevention, diagnosis, treatment, and management of disease. Pharmacoeconomics thus provides information critical to the optimal allocation of health care resources. The field encompasses experts of health economics, risk analysis, technology assessment, clinical evaluation, epidemiology, decision sciences and health services research.

## EXPLANATION

Pharmacoeconomics is a collection of descriptive and analytic techniques for evaluating pharmaceutical interventions in the health care system. Pharmaco-economic techniques include cost minimization, cost effectiveness, cost utility, cost benefit, cost of illness, cost consequence, and any other economic analytic technique that provides valuable information to health care decision makers for the allocation of scarce resources. Pharmacoeconomics is often referred to as health economics (*see terms:* Cost-Benefit Analysis, Cost-Consequence Analysis, Cost-Effectiveness Analysis, Cost-Minimization Analysis, Cost-Utility Analysis, Health Economics) or health outcomes research, especially when it includes nonpharmaceutical courses of therapy or preventive strategies, such as surgical interventions or screening techniques.

## VALUE AND USE

Several potential uses for pharmacoeconomic analyses are in pharmaceutical reimbursement, price negotiations, formulary discussions, clinical practice guide-line developments, and communications to prescribing physicians. In recent years, pharmacoeconomics has grown rapidly because its core subject, cost-effectiveness analysis, is easy to apply and has powerful applications for health care decision making in both the public and private sectors. Recent research from the Tufts Center for the Study of Drug Development suggests that the demand for phar-macoeconomic analyses conducted by the pharmaceutical industry is likely to grow substantially from the present spending (average 1% of pharmaceutical research and development cost) in the near future. In Australia and Canada, the acceptance of new chemical entities in the national or provincial formularies depends on pharmacoeconomic studies. Different countries have different approaches to making pricing and reimbursement decisions using formal phar-macoeconomic evaluations. In a recent study based on nine European countries (Finland, France, Germany, Norway, Austria, The Netherlands, Portugal, Spain, and the United Kingdom), one-third of all respondents (government agencies, physicians, hospital pharmacists, hospital managers, sickness funds, and the pharmaceutical industry) across all countries stated that they have used results from health economics studies for decision making (Hoffman 2000). In the United States, pharmacoeconomic analyses are not required for the submission of a new drug to the Food and Drug Administration (FDA). However, the potential value of pharmacoeconomics in drug coverage decisions by private and public health plans is promising. In a recent survey, 88% of the 24 managed care decision makers from 15 companies across the United States indicated that pharmacoeconomic information is useful. Managed care plans are increasingly requiring or encouraging the submission of pharmacoeconomic information (sometimes in "dossier" format) by pharmaceutical companies seeking cover-age of or reimbursement for new therapies.

ISSUES

The credibility of pharmacoeconomics lies in developing studies in accordance with generally applicable standards of analysis and interpretation. Then users can translate pharmacoeconomic research findings into practices to ensure that decision makers allocate scarce health care resources wisely, fairly, and efficiently. Several groups in the United States (an expert panel commissioned by the United States Public Health Service, Center for Disease Control and Prevention; and the Division of Drug Marketing, Advertising, and Communication [DDMAC] of the FDA) have developed guidelines for proper conduct of pharmacoeconomic studies. The Academy of Managed Care Pharmacy has developed guidelines for formulary submission (AMCP 2002). This guideline contains extensive information on which pharmacoeconomic data should be included for consideration of drug coverage decisions. Individual countries, including Australia, Canada, Italy, Spain, The Netherlands, Switzerland, Germany, France, and the United Kingdom have developed their own sets of guidelines. The Pharmaceutical Research and Manufacturers of America (PhRMA) also developed a set of voluntary principles to guide industry members in conducting pharmacoeconomic studies that minimize bias and ensure transparency. The future success of pharmacoeconomic analyses relies on the continued accumulation and dissemination of robust information that can be utilized by different users under different circumstances.

BIBLIOGRAPHY

Academy of Managed Care Pharmacy (AMCP). Format for Formulary Submissions Version 2.0. October 2002. http://www.fmcpnet.org/data/resource/formatv20.pdf. Accessed August 27, 2003.

Fry RN, Avey SG, Sullivan SD. The academy of managed care pharmacy format for formulary submissions: An evolving standard—A foundation for managed care pharmacy task force report. *Value Health* 2003;6:505–521.

Grizzle AJ, Olson BM, Motheral BR, et al. Therapeutic value: who decides? *Pharmaceutical Executive*. 2000;84–90.

Hoffman C, Graf von der Schulenburg JM. The influence of economic evaluation studies on decision making: a European survey. *The EUROMET Group Health Policy*. 2000;52:179–192.

Pashos CL, Klein EG, Wanke LA. *ISPOR LEXICON First Edition*. Princeton: International Society for Pharmacoeconomics and Outcomes Research; 1998.

# Pharmacoepidemiology

Efficacy
Effectiveness
Channeling

BRIEF DEFINITION

In **pharmacoepidemiology**, the use, effects, and outcomes of drug treatment are studied from an epidemiological perspective—that is, from a population perspective (*see term:* Drug Safety).

## Explanation

Pharmacoepidemiology combines knowledge from pharmacology and therapeutics with methods and reasoning from epidemiology (*see term:* Epidemiology). The interest is focused on population groups or the population as a whole and not merely on clinical settings. One area of interest is the extent of drug use in the population and factors that are of importance for the prescribing and use of drugs (*see term:* Drug Use Evaluation). Pharmacoepidemiology deals with both positive outcomes—such as a better therapeutical effect, a better prognosis, a higher life expectancy, and an increased quality of life—and negative outcomes—such as adverse reactions, misuse, and dependence.

## Value and Use

Different epidemiological designs are used in pharmacoepidemiology. Information on sales statistics—only available on the aggregate level—is used to follow use of drugs over time and to make comparisons between countries and regions (drug-utilization studies). Cross-sectional studies are used to study differences in use of drugs and related matters at a certain point in time. Case-control studies and cohort studies are employed to analyze effects and outcomes of the use of drugs in clinical practice. Randomized clinical trials are another important source of information on the effect of a drug treatment. The advantage of randomized clinical trials is that they study the outcome under controlled circumstances and with minimization of biases. However, the trials are limited in terms of the number of patients studied and length of exposure, and they are rarely representative of the target population. The effect of drug treatment in controlled circumstances in clinical trials is termed **efficacy** of drug use (*see terms:* Clinical Trial, Drug Efficacy), while the effect of drug treatment in clinical practice, in natural or "real-world" settings, is termed **effectiveness** (*see terms:* Drug Efficacy, Observational Study). Another important aspect of pharmacoepidemiology is the safety of drugs and the study of adverse reactions to drug treatment (*see terms:* Drug Research and Development, Drug Safety). Both analytical studies and spontaneous reporting systems are used.

Pharmacoepidemiology conducted before marketing approval can improve safety monitoring by organizing data resources (both internal and external) and anticipating potential issues in advance in order to answer questions as rapidly as possible. Pharmacoepidemiology conducted after marketing approval of a drug can supplement information from premarketing studies, leading to higher precision in the risk estimate of known adverse effects. Pharmacoepidemiology can also provide, from postmarketing drug surveillance studies, information not available from premarketing studies such as previously undetected adverse and beneficial effects, including uncommon effects and delayed effects, patterns of drug utilization, effects of drug overdoses, and economic implications of drug use. In addition, pharmacoepidemiology can lead to reassurances about drug safety and help to fulfill ethical and legal obligations. The aim of pharmacoepidemiology is to achieve a safer and more rational use of drugs for patients and for the society at large. In pharmacoepidemiology during the last decade, more and more interest has focused on patient-reported outcomes such as health-related quality of life. At the same time pharmacoepidemiology is increasingly being regarded as an important tool in pharmacoeconomics.

## ISSUES

There are many examples in pharmacoepidemiology of controversies concerning the outcome of a certain drug treatment. Discussions on causality, therefore, are important. Controversies exist about the strength of certain associations as well as about the detection of adverse reactions. Also subject to controversy in pharmacoepidemiological studies are the drug or placebo used for comparison, the dosage used, the patient or population group selected for the study, and so on. There are particular problems with confounding and bias (*see terms:* Clinical Trial – Study Bias, Epidemiology).

Compliance (*see term:* Compliance) with drug regimens is an area of considerable interest, which has not been the subject of many epidemiological studies so far. Another aspect is **channeling:** when a new drug is introduced, there may be a tendency toward channeling (i.e., selecting) patients who are not doing well on the older drug for treatment with the new drug. Thus, patients who receive the new drug could have a worse prognosis as compared to the patients who remain on the older treatment.

Pharmacoepidemiological studies are sometimes performed with the use of drug sales statistics and computerized databases on disease frequency or vital statistics. There are several studies in which ecological correlations between sales statistics on drugs and the frequency of such things as suicides and cancer incidences have been conducted. One major problem with such studies, when data is only available on the aggregate level, is ecological fallacy. Also, several problems have been pointed out with respect to the use of computerized databases with data on an individual level. Some researchers claim that there is not enough relevant medical and other information available in the databases to control for important confounders. One much-discussed source of bias is confounding by indication, in which it is difficult to separate the effect of the drug on the outcome studied from the effect of the disease for which the drug is given. Another issue being discussed is the representativeness of the databases used in research.

## BIBLIOGRAPHY

Hartzema AG, Porta MS, Tilson HH, eds. *Pharmacoepidemiology: An Introduction.* 3rd ed. Cincinnati, Ohio: Harvey Whitney Books Company; 1998.
Strom BL, ed. *Pharmacoepidemiology.* 3rd ed. New York: John Wiley & Sons; 2000.

# Pharmacogenomics
Pharmacogenetics

## BRIEF DEFINITION

**Pharmacogenomics** is the application of genomics to pharmaceutical research using genome studies to identify genes that account for differences in different individuals (*see term:* Gene Therapy). Based on either genetic testing for predisposition to a disease or variation in response to a therapeutic intervention (i.e., a medication, or radiation therapy), pharmacogenomics has the potential to personalize medical therapies.

**Pharmacogenetics** determines what the right medicine is for the individual patient based upon the small genetic variations that can be measured by genetic testing of a single nucleotide polymorphism (SNP). An SNP is a common variation that occurs in human DNA at a frequency of one every 1,000 base pair. These variations can be familial or occur de novo.

EXPLANATION

Genes produce proteins. Variation among genes and their protein products can help us understand risk for specific conditions, the natural history of health conditions, and potential differences in response to specific therapies. Pharmacogenomics links our understanding of genetics with pharmaceuticals to more appropriately target therapies. For example, the response of Alzheimer's patients to tacrine, a cholinomimetic drug, is reduced among those who have the subtype ApoE4 (Fink and Collins 2000).

VALUE AND USE

The explosion of information about the human genome and human genetics has created enormous potential opportunity for targeting prevention and treatment. Genetic information can be used to understand individuals' risk for specific conditions and likelihood of benefit or harm from specific therapies. Pharmacogenomics and pharmacogenetics are closely related concepts. They involve identification of specific genomes, which can be used to develop and target therapies based on understanding of specific mechanisms and variations in response.

Matching patients and drugs based on the patient's genetic characteristics may decrease the variation in response to drugs, improve their effectiveness, and enhance safety.

ISSUES

Genetics has historically been laden with social and ethical issues. Among these are

- Labeling of individuals and potential risks associated with knowledge of risk of conditions (e.g., job discrimination, privacy, and insurability);
- Careful counseling and consents that may be required for use of pharmacogenetic treatments and associated testing;
- Cost of development and implementation: pharmacogenetic treatments are potentially costly. On the development side, therapies may be targeted to small numbers of individuals at specific risk, which may limit use of drugs. This leads to costly development on a per-patient basis. Conversely, better targeting of drugs may increase their value to the individual patient—for example, by assuring that patients are likely to benefit or reducing risk of harms. Associated laboratory testing to identify those with

specific genetic characteristics may also increase cost. The trade-offs among these costs and benefits remain to be elucidated in practice;
- Availability of potentially costly therapies; and
- Trial design that may need to incorporate understanding of genetic variation in patient selection.

BIBLIOGRAPHY

American Medical Association (AMA). Pharmacogenomics. http://www.ama-assn.org/ama/pub/category/2306.html. Accessed August 28, 2003.

Fink L, Collins FS. The human genome project: evolving status and emerging opportunities for disease prevention. In: Khoury MJ, Burke W, Thomson EJ, eds. *Genetics and Public Health in the 21st Century.* New York: Oxford University Press; 2000.

# Pharmacokinetics

Biopharmaceutics
Bioavailability
Clinical Pharmacokinetics
Pharmacodynamics
Therapeutic Drug Monitoring
Bioequivalence

## BRIEF DEFINITION

**Pharmacokinetics** is the study of the time course of what the body does to a drug (absorption, distribution, elimination) in contrast to pharmacodynamics, which is the study of what the drug does to the body.

## EXPLANATION

The study of the interrelationships of various physiochemical properties of drugs such as absorption, bioavailability, distribution, metabolism, and excretion (ADME) is called **biopharmaceutics**. **Bioavailability** is the fraction or percent of an administered drug that reaches systemic circulation. Many factors such as rate of absorption, route of administration, dosage form, gastrointestinal wall metabolism, and hepatic first pass metabolism can affect a drug's bioavailability. The further study of these biopharmaceutic properties as they relate to drug concentration over time is termed pharmacokinetics. The application of these pharmacokinetic principles to direct patient care is termed **clinical pharmacokinetics**. **Pharmacodynamics** refers to the relationship between drug concentration at the site of action and the resulting effect, including the time course and intensity of therapeutic and adverse effects. Lastly, the use of pharmacokinetic and pharmacodynamic principles to individualize a specific drug dosing and monitoring plan is termed **therapeutic drug monitoring**.

   **Bioequivalence** compares the pharmacokinetic characteristics of two chemically similar drug products (pharmaceutical equivalents). For instance, a generic drug can be considered bioequivalent to the branded product if the manufacturer is able to prove that it displays the same concentration-time characteristics as the brand product within a statistical certainty (*see term:* Drug).

## VALUE AND USE

Drug concentration versus time curves, as shown in the figure, can be used to characterize various "kinetic" processes. Mathematical models can be used to calculate various pharmacokinetic variables such as peak drug concentration, time-to-peak drug concentration, rate of drug elimination, volume of distribution, dosing interval, etc. Specific equations can then be written that apply these models to various drug dosing scenarios in order to determine more accurately the amount of drug necessary to achieve a therapeutic concentration resulting in the desired therapeutic effect, while avoiding both subtherapeutic and supra-

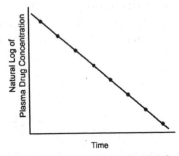

therapeutic or toxic drug concentrations. Drug dosing can then be individualized for such patient variables as renal or hepatic insufficiency, body weight, age, sex, and disease states. This process results in a more economic use of drug product and hospital resources. The amount and therefore the cost of drugs used can be optimized, thus maximizing attainment of desired clinical outcomes.

An example of the utility of bioequivalence data is in the use of FDA-rated generic products as a substitute for more expensive branded products. Manufacturers of generic drugs have to submit human pharmacokinetic data to the FDA in order to prove that their drug is bioequivalent to the branded product. The FDA will then grant that product its "AB bioequivalence rating" (i.e., approved generic) thus allowing for the legal substitution of that product. Health insurance plans also use bioequivalence data when determining reimbursement rates for multisource drugs. FDA-approved bioequivalence data is found in the FDA publication *Approved Drug Products with Therapeutic Equivalence Evaluations* (also known as the Orange Book).

## ISSUES

Pharmacokinetic and bioequivalence data can be used to make econo-therapeutic decisions regarding drug formularies (*see term:* Drug Formulary) and appropriate drug usage. An active institutional clinical pharmacokinetics program is a valuable aid in working with medical staffs to reduce unnecessary drug costs while also optimizing drug usage. This clinical activity can be used to support the institution's efforts at gaining medical staff approval for controlling overall drug usage and expense. Physicians in some countries have learned to use the clinical pharmacy department as a consulting service to calculate correct drug dosage and to monitor for both desired outcomes and untoward effects. In the United States, the Joint Commission on Accreditation of Health Care Organizations (JCAHO) now requires hospitals to document that they have an active drug dosing and monitoring policy for certain drugs having a narrow therapeutic index. Examples include the aminoglycosides, vancomycin, phenytoin, and warfarin.

BIBLIOGRAPHY

Bauer LA. *Applied Clinical Pharmacokinetics.* New York: McGraw-Hill; 2001.

DiPiro JT, Spruill WJ. *Concepts in Clinical Pharmacokinetics.* 3rd ed. Bethesda, Md: American Society of Health-System Pharmacists; 2002.

European Agency for the Evaluation of Medicinal Products: http://www.emea.eu.int/. Accessed March 23, 2003.

Food and Drug Administration: Approved Drug Products with Therapeutic Equivalence Evalutions. April 2002. http://www.fda.gov/cder/orange/adp.htm. Accessed March 23, 2003.

# Pharmacy Benefit Management Organization (PBM)

BRIEF DEFINITION

A **pharmacy benefit management organization (PBM)** is a company that administers the pharmacy benefit on behalf of employers, managed care organizations, and other third party payers, with the stated goal of making prescription drugs more affordable and safer.

EXPLANATION

To administer the benefits, PBMs process pharmacy claims, create networks of retail pharmacies, develop formularies, negotiate discounts from retail pharmacies and pharmaceutical manufacturers, offer mail pharmacy services, provide consultative services on pharmacy benefit design, and offer various clinical and safety programs, such as drug utilization review.

VALUE AND USE

A PBM can reduce the costs associated with pharmaceuticals by providing services for third party payers that may otherwise be too difficult or costly to administer. A single PBM may have several clients wanting similar services and can usually provide these services at a lower cost than if their clients implemented them independently. In addition, a PBM usually represents a large number of patients and thus purchasing power, allowing them to negotiate better prices from community pharmacies and rebates from pharmaceutical manufacturers. Savings through the use of a PBM have been estimated at 2–27% of the pharmacy benefit costs. A PBM also helps to make prescription drug use safer by providing timely warnings to pharmacists about possible harm from inappropriate medications. Because a PBM processes patients' claims from all pharmacies, PBM is in the unique position of being able to identify drug–drug interactions, overdosing, and other potential drug problems. After prescriptions are dispensed, PBMs continue to identify potential safety risks and to notify physicians.

ISSUES

The relationships and incentives that a PBM has established with pharmaceutical manufacturers and retail pharmacies, including ownership, has been an area of ongoing concern and evaluation by US governmental agencies and patient advocacy groups that are concerned about PBM practices and their alignment with patient health goals and product promotional regulations.

While PBMs have reported cost-savings on pharmaceutical budgets, the support for these statements has relied heavily on PBM-supplied data. There is limited evidence on whether cost-saving measures adversely or positively affect patient quality of care.

Several barriers exist to conducting research designed to determine the true effects of a PBM's interventions on the health of patients and the cost of care, such as the proprietary nature of data, the lack of meaningful baseline measures, the complex delivery of health care, and the difficulty in combining prescription claims data with clinical outcome.

BIBLIOGRAPHY

Kreling DH, Lipton HL, Collins TC, Hertz KC. *Assessment of the impact of pharmacy benefit managers: Final report to the Health Care Financing Administration.* Publ No. PB97-103683. Springfield, Va: National Technical Information Service; 1996.

Lipton HL, Kreling DH, Collins T, Hertz KC. Pharmacy benefit management companies: Dimensions of performance. *Annu Rev Public Health.* 1999;20:361–401.

Saikami D. Financial risk management of pharmacy benefits. *Am J Health-Syst Pharm.* 1997;54:2207–2212.

US General Accounting Office. *Pharmacy benefit managers: FEHBP plans satisfied with savings and services, but retail pharmacies have concerns.* GAO/HEHS-97-47. Washington, DC: US Government Printing Office; 1997.

US Office of Inspector General, Department of Health and Human Services. *Experiences of health maintenance organizations with pharmacy benefit management companies.* Publ. No. OEI-01-95-00110. Washington, DC: US Government Printing Office; 1997.

# Predictive Value
## Positive Predictive Value
## Negative Predictive Value
## Sensitivity
## Specificity

BRIEF DEFINITION

In screening and diagnostic tests, the probability that a person with a positive test is a true positive (i.e., has the disease), is referred to as the **predictive value** of a positive test, whereas the predictive value of a negative test is the probability that the person with a negative test does not have the disease. Predictive value is related to the sensitivity and specificity of the test and the prevalence of the disease in the population tested.

EXPLANATION

The predictive value is clearly an important public health consideration. In effect we are asking: if test results are positive, what is the probability that the person has the disease? This is called the **positive predictive value** of the test. In other words, what proportion of patients who test positive actually have the disease in question? To calculate the predictive value, we divide the number of true positives by the total number who tested positive (true-positives plus false-positives). A parallel question can be asked relating to negative tests: if the test result is negative, what is the probability that this patient does not have the disease? This is called the **negative predictive value** of the test. It is calculated by dividing the number of true negatives by all those who tested negative (true-negatives plus false-negatives). The **sensitivity** of the test is defined as the ability of the test to identify correctly those who truly have the disease, which in other words is estimated by dividing the number of true positives by the sum of true positive and false negatives. The **specificity** of the test is defined as the ability of the test to identify correctly those who do not have the disease. Specificity is obtained by dividing the number of true negatives by the sum of true negatives and false positives, as shown in the table.

Comparison of the Results of a Dichotomous Test with Disease Status

| Test Result | Population | |
|---|---|---|
| | With disease | Without disease |
| Positive | True positive (TP) | False positive (FP) |
| Negative | False negative (FN) | True negative (TN) |

Using these terms, the following metrics can be defined.

$$Sensitivity = TP/(TP + FN)$$
$$Specificity = TN/(TN + FP)$$
$$Positive\ predictive\ value = TP/(TP + FP)$$
$$Negative\ predictive\ value = TN/(TN + FN)$$

## VALUE AND USE

The accuracy of diagnostic tests is evaluated in terms of their sensitivity, specificity, and predictive values. These values are commonly used in cost-benefit analysis to assess the efficiency of diagnostic tests, screening and vaccination programs, and other public health interventions. (*See term:* Likelihood Ratio)

## ISSUES

The sensitivity and specificity of a test and the prevalence of the disease in the population tested affect the positive predictive value of the test. The figure shows the relation between disease prevalence and predictive values in a test with a sensitivity of 95% and a specificity of 95%. Most of the gains in the predictive value occur with increases in prevalence at the lowest rates of disease population. The higher the prevalence, the higher the predictive value. This has significant economic consequences. A screening program is most productive and efficient if it is directed to a high-risk target population. Screening a total population for a relatively infrequent disease can be wasteful of resources and may yield few previously undetected cases for the amount of effort involved. How-

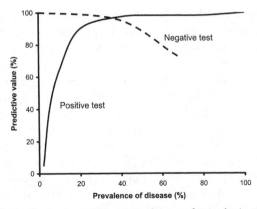

Relationship between disease prevalence and negative/positive
predictive value in a test with 95% sensitivity and 95% specificity
Reprinted from *Mausner and Bahn Epidemiology: An Introductory Text.* Mausner
JS, Kramer S (authors), p. 221. © 1985, with permission from Elsevier.

ever, if a high-risk subset can be identified and the screening can be directed to
that group, the program is likely to be more productive. This relation also demonstrates that the results of any test must be interpreted in the context of the
prevalence of the disease in the population from which the subject originates.

### BIBLIOGRAPHY
Gordis L. *Epidemiology.* 2nd ed. Philadelphia: WB Saunders Company; 2000.
Health Decision Strategy. www.healthstrategy.com
Mausner JS, Kramer S. *Mausner and Bahn Epidemiology: An Introductory Text.* Philadelphia: WB
Saunders; 1985.

# Prevalence
Point Prevalence
Period Prevalence
Lifetime Prevalence
Prevalence Odds

### BRIEF DEFINITION
**Prevalence** is defined as the proportion of a population that is affected by a disease under study at a given point in time.

### EXPLANATION
Prevalence can be seen as a dichotomous measurement of a disease state (having the disease or not) at a hypothetical point in time for a defined population.
The numerator reports the group of individuals having the disease under study
at a given point in time. Prevalence rates are easily measured through cross-

sectional studies performed at a certain point in time in a well-defined population. A prevalence rate will result in a **point prevalence** estimate, which could have a different value from a **period prevalence** estimate. In the latter, both the numerator and the denominator are calculated during a period or an interval. If the interval is, for instance, one year, the prevalence number will be a compound measure including the prevalence at the starting point of the observation period plus the new cases occurring over the next year plus the recurrences during the same time period. The denominator is the stable total population present during the period of observation. Period prevalence is sometimes preferred over point prevalence measuring for chronic conditions in which disease onset is difficult to define without a certain period of observation. Classical examples are arthritis and mental disorders. A variant of the period prevalence is the **lifetime prevalence**, which is the proportion of a population that has a history of a given disease at a certain point in time or who ever has been a case with the disease under study. Therefore, the numerator contains the individuals that have the disease under study plus those individuals that were previously cured of the disease plus the individuals in remission. This measure could only be obtained retrospectively and must be estimated by using subject recall and/or medical records. A special measure sometimes used is the **prevalence odds**. It is the ratio of the probability of having the disease under study divided by the probability of not having the disease at a certain point in time within a defined population.

## VALUE AND USE

Prevalence data are often used to indicate the amount of a disease problem or its burden within a defined population at a given point in time. This is particularly useful for chronic conditions in order to determine and plan workload, resource use, and further investments to be done. Also, when monitoring and controlling chronic conditions, it may be helpful to have access to accurate prevalence data over time measured through cross-sectional surveys of the population. This is much cheaper than developing longitudinal surveillance or cohort studies. Prevalence studies will therefore be an integral part of cost of illness studies where not only the burden but also the cost of dealing with the disease under study is reported.

There is an interrelationship between incidence (I), prevalence (P), and the average duration of the disease (D) in a stable situation and assuming that the prevalence of the disease in the population is low, i.e. less than 0.1.

$$P = I \times D$$

## ISSUES

Prevalence data are different from incidence data in which the numerator and the denominator have different definitions and will result in different values (*see term:* Incidence). Incidence data are essential for etiologic studies and are direct indicators of risk of the disease under study, whereas prevalence data have some important limitations in that respect. They tend to produce a biased picture of a disease with acute and chronic episodes toward the chronic condition that prevails. Using single cross-sectional prevalence studies to determine incidence and/or risk factors has severe limitations since at least two measurements are needed to assess both values. It is therefore appropriate that besides measuring the prevalence of a disease under study, researchers should separately collect and adequately report incidence data.

## BIBLIOGRAPHY

Kleinbaum DG, Kupper LL, Morgenstein H. *Epidemiologic Research—Principles and Quantitative Methods.* Belmont, Calif.: Lifetime Learning Publications; 1982.

Mausner J, Kramer S. *Epidemiology—An Introductory Text.* 2nd ed. Philadelphia: WB Saunders Company; 1984.

Rothman KJ, Greenland S. *Modern Epidemiology.* 2nd ed. Philadelphia: Lippincott-Raven; 1997.

# Public Health

## BRIEF DEFINITION

**Public health** activities are what society does to assure the conditions for people to be healthy. The term encompasses the activities undertaken within the formal structure of government and the associated efforts of private and voluntary organizations and individuals (Institute of Medicine, 1988).

## EXPLANATION

Public health is

> one of the efforts organized by society to protect, promote, and restore the people's health. It is a combination of sciences, skills, and beliefs that is directed to the maintenance and improvement of the health of all the people through collective or social actions. The programs, services, and institutions involved emphasize the prevention of disease and the health needs of the population as a whole. Public health activities change with changing technology and social values, but the goals remain the same: to reduce the amount of disease, premature death, and disease-produced discomfort and disability in the population. Public health is thus a social institution, a discipline and practice. (Last 2001)

The core functions of public health are categorized as

Assessment—understanding the determinants and distribution of disease and injury, and the health and economic consequences of those conditions.

Policy—Policy development requires an understanding not only about the determinants and distribution of health conditions and their consequences, but effective means for improving those conditions. Based on the needs and evidence of what works and recognizing issues of equity and feasibility, policy-makers are responsible for developing and implementing strategies for meeting those needs. These might include regulatory, educational, programmatic, guidelines and standards, research, or other strategies.

Assurance—Government, in particular, is responsible for assuring the availability of public health services to everyone.

It is estimated that 95% of health dollars are spent on personal health care, leaving the remainder for population health activities. These include setting and monitoring community-wide standards (e.g., for health care, the environment), assuring safe and healthful environments, operating programs to support healthy lifestyles, identifying and responding to public health threats (e.g., outbreaks, terrorism, emerging health problems), assuring the availability of health care services, and preventing and controlling health problems.

## VALUE AND USE

Public health is a joint responsibility of government, the health care system, employers, the media, academia, private and voluntary organizations, and the community. It is the broad framework under which the health care system functions.

## ISSUES

There are many important issues in public health:

- Healthy People 2010, a report of the Office of Disease Prevention and Health Promotion, US Department of Health and Human Services, sets out health objectives for the United States. These have been embraced by the organized public health sector, although not by the health care system in general. There is a keen need to have shared goals, objectives, and efforts.
- Health behaviors (e.g., physical activity, eating, tobacco use, sexual behaviors) remain the largest contributor to adverse health in this country. Better strategies for improving these behaviors and programs to implement them are needed.
- There are large disparities in health within the United States and even larger disparities around the world.
- Global health issues affect the developed world. Infectious diseases remain globally important (e.g., malaria, acute respiratory and gastrointestinal illness) and can readily be imported (e.g., resistant tuberculosis, West Nile Virus).
- Public heath is responsible for controlling bioterrorism threats.

## BIBLIOGRAPHY

Last JM. *A Dictionary of Epidemiology.* 4th ed. New York: Oxford University Press; 2001.
Institute of Medicine. *The Future of Public Health.* National Academy Press: Washington, DC; 1988.

# Quality-Adjusted Life Year (QALY)

## BRIEF DEFINITION

A quality-adjusted life year (QALY) is a universal health outcome measure applicable to all individuals and all diseases, thereby enabling comparisons across diseases and across programs. A QALY combines, in a single measure, gains or losses in both quantity of life (mortality) and quality of life (morbidity).

## EXPLANATION

Quality-adjusted life years are life years adjusted by a preference-based quality weight. The quality weight is measured on a preference scale, usually a utility scale, where full health has a score of 1.0, being dead has a score of 0.0, and states worse than being dead can have negative scores (*see term:* Utility Measurement).

For example, if an individual lived for 10 years in full health, followed by 10 years in a health state with a quality weight of 0.5, followed by death, the individual would have achieved $10 \times 1.0 + 10 \times 0.5 = 15$ QALYs. Now suppose with a new treatment the same individual could live for 10 years in full health, 6 years in a health state valued at 0.8, 6 years in a state valued at 0.5, followed by death. In this second scenario, the individual would have achieved $10 \times 1.0 + 6 \times 0.8 + 6 \times 0.5 = 17.8$ QALYs. Note that although the treatment created only 2.0 additional life years (LYs), it created 2.8 additional QALYs. Of course, this will not always be the case. Sometimes the number of QALYs gained will be less than the number of LYs gained. The important point is that the number of QALYs gained captures both the change in quantity of life and the change in quality of life, and the number will, in general, be different from the number of LYs gained.

For simplicity, the above example ignored discounting. In practice, it would be normal to "discount" the future years by an appropriate discount rate (*see term:* Discounting).

The quality weights for QALYs must be preference-based and must be measured on an interval scale on which full health has a score of 1.0 and being dead has a score of 0.0. To be preference-based, the quality weights must represent the preferences of individuals for the relevant health states as measured with appropriate preference measurement instruments. Such instruments include standard gamble, time trade-off, Health Utilities Index, EuroQol EQ-5D, and quality of well-being (*see terms:* EuroQol, Health Utilities Index, Utility).

VALUE AND USE

The QALY approach is widely used. It is the preferred outcome measure for cost-utility analysis because it captures changes in both quantity of life and quality of life, it is universally applicable to all patients and all diseases, and it can be linked to formal utility theory (*see term:* Cost-Utility Analysis). QALYs are the preferred outcome measure identified in any of the country-specific guidelines for economic evaluation that specify a preferred measure.

QALYs are also used in clinical studies that have no economic component. QALYs enable disparate clinical outcomes like mortality, morbidity, and adverse events to be aggregated into a summary measure that reflects the preferences associated with the different outcomes.

QALYs are beginning to be used in routine clinical practice. Some clinics, for example, routinely collect data using the Health Utilities Index and use the data both for patient management as well as for research.

QALYs are increasingly being used in population health. In this field QALYs are used to monitor, report, and compare the health of communities, provinces, and even countries. The QALY approach is used to calculate quality-adjusted life expectancies by age and sex for each jurisdiction. Canada has been the leading country in developing these methods. The World Health Organization is now promoting this approach worldwide, although it calls its version disability-adjusted life years (DALYs) (*see term:* Disability-Adjusted Life Year).

QALYs are particularly well suited for long-term health outcomes. They are more problematic when applied to very short-term outcomes—as, for example, the use of anesthesia for dental work. The value of such short-term outcomes may be better measured using other approaches such as contingent valuation.

ISSUES

The QALY concept requires that the quality weights be based on preferences, but does not specify whose preferences should count. In particular, should the preferences come from the informed general public (community preferences) or should they come from patients? Are different sources of preferences required for different types of applications? Although this is still an area of debate, the current recommendation for cost-utility analyses is that community preferences are the most relevant, although patients' preferences, if different, should also be investigated and discussed. On the other hand, for population health applications there is no debate; community preferences are preferred.

The QALY approach is indifferent to whether the QALY gain comes from a small gain for a large number of individuals or a large gain for a small number of people. Although the preference measurements implicitly take that trade-off into account, some researchers debate whether the result is appropriate. They argue that more weight should be given to large gains for few people, particularly when the gains are life-saving.

A healthy-year equivalent (HYE) has been proposed as an alternative to a QALY (*see term:* Healthy-Years Equivalent). After much debate in the literature, the conclusion appears to be that the first stage of the HYE measurement procedure produces a more accurate QALY than the traditional QALY approach but at a greatly increased measurement burden. The second stage of the HYE measurement procedure produces the actual HYE, and this may sometimes be useful as a communication tool. However, if the goal is to produce the HYE result, it is simpler to bypass the two-stage measurement procedure and use an equivalent one-stage procedure (*see term:* Healthy-Years Equivalent).

One of the major advantages of the QALY approach is its universality. It is applicable to all patients and all diseases, and thus produces a level playing field for making comparisons across programs. However, this advantage is compromised if different sources of quality weights are used in different QALY applications. Unfortunately, we know that different utility measurement instruments give systematically different results (*see term:* Utility Measurement). Thus, for example, a QALY calculated with the Health Utilities Index may not be directly comparable with one calculated with the EuroQol EQ-5D. Further research is required to determine the extent of the problem and, if needed, to suggest possible solutions like conversion curves.

BIBLIOGRAPHY

Canadian Coordinating Office for Health Technology Assessment. *Guidelines for Economic Evaluation of Pharmaceuticals: Canada.* 2nd ed. Ottawa: CCOHTA; 1997.

Drummond MF, O'Brien BJ, Stoddart GL, Torrance GW. *Methods for the Economic Evaluation of Health Care Programmes.* 2nd ed. Oxford, UK: Oxford University Press; 1997.

Gold MR, Siegel JE, Russell LB, Weinstein MC. *Cost-Effectiveness in Health and Medicine.* New York: Oxford University Press; 1996.

## Quality Assurance (QA)
Continuous Quality Assurance (CQA)
Practice Profiling

BRIEF DEFINITION

**Quality assurance** is formal set of activities that aim to measure and improve the quality of health care services provided, including medical, administrative, and other support services (*see term:* Quality of Care).

EXPLANATION

Quality assurance includes an initial assessment phase and follow-up actions to remedy any deficiencies identified through the assessment. **Continuous quality assurance (CQA)** is a dynamic quality assurance process based on the notion that quality of health care services can be improved and that such improvement is continuous and based on monitoring performance and identifying improvement opportunities.

## VALUE AND USE

Indicative of the national effort to promote quality assurance for health insurance plans is the development of "report cards" by the National Committee for Quality Assurance (NCQA, 2003), an accreditation organization recognized by the managed care industry in the United States. NCQA publishes a widely used standardized quality measurement tool, the Health Plan Employer Data and Information Set (HEDIS). Its stated purpose is to systematically collect and publish health plans' quality information to help employers and consumers make better decisions. HEDIS measures are based primarily on analyses of administrative data sets and tend usually to measure process, rather than outcomes, related to the delivery of appropriate preventive care and care for selected disease states. For example, current HEDIS measures include rates of immunization of infants and adolescents, flu shots for at-risk adults, cervical cancer screening, treatment of otitis media, asthma treatment for children and adults, smoking cessation efforts, and the assessment of functional status for elderly patients.

In addition, quality assurance can be applied to measure and improve physicians' performance. **Practice profiling** is an important and increasingly common way of evaluating and improving physician behavior through benchmarking a physician's practice pattern and comparing it with his or her peer group or peer-reviewed guidelines. This has been done both by government agencies and by private organizations.

## ISSUES

The majority of current health plan or physician performance measures, such as HEDIS, are derived from administrative data and offer little insight into health outcomes associated with treating serious illnesses. Problems also arise due to the use of different operational definitions in data collection and the lack of appropriate risk adjustment. An alternative method of standardized surveys is proposed that may overcome the current limitations, provide outcome rather than process data, and help develop interventions to improve quality.

## BIBLIOGRAPHY

Chassin MR. Quality of health care, III: improving the quality of care. *N Engl J Med.* 1996; 335:1060–1062.

Institute of Medicine. *Medicare: A Strategy for Quality Assurance.* Washington, DC: National Academy Press; 1990.

National Committee for Quality Assurance (NCQA). http://www.ncqa.org. Accessed January 6, 2003.

# Quality of Care

## BRIEF DEFINITION

A 1990 Institute of Medicine (IOM) report defined **quality of care** as "the degree to which health services for individuals and populations increase the likelihood of desired health outcomes and are consistent with current professional knowledge" (*see term:* Quality Assurance [QA]).

## EXPLANATION

There are generally three dimensions of quality of care: effectiveness of care, access to care, and patient satisfaction with care. Quality of care problems can also be categorized into two broad groups: undertreatment and overtreatment. Examples for undertreatment include the use of beta-blockers and angiotensin-converting enzyme (ACE) inhibitors for patients with chronic heart failure and the use of statins for postmyocardial infarction patients. An example for over-treatment is the over prescribing of antibiotics for children with ear aches. Inherent in determining the quality of care is a strong recognition of the importance of the peer-review process in identifying and updating quality of care measures.

## VALUE AND USE

The construction of a framework to measure quality of care generally involves five elements: (1) the purpose of quality measurement, (2) the patient population, (3) the timing of measurement, (4) the source of patient information, and (5) the setting(s) in which care is to be measured. Quality of care measures are often established through a peer-review process by professional societies and often governmental agencies. For example, the National Cholesterol Education Program regularly reviews and updates the diagnostic and treatment guidelines for high blood cholesterol based on risk levels of coronary artery disease.

## ISSUES

Currently many quality of care measures are process instead of health outcome measures. This is mainly due to the lack of appropriate risk adjustment methods for many diseases. Cautions should be taken in interpreting and publishing those quality of care measures without appropriate risk adjustment so that physicians or hospitals treating more high-risk patients are not incorrectly labeled as low-quality providers.

## BIBLIOGRAPHY

Blumenthal D. Quality of health care, I: Quality of care—What is it? *N Engl J Med.* 1996;335:891–894.

Brook RH, McGlynn EA, Cleary PD. Quality of health care, II: Measuring quality of care. *N Engl J Med.* 1996;335:966–970.

Institute of Medicine. *Medicare: A Strategy for Quality Assurance.* Washington, DC: National Academy Press; 1990.

# Quality of Well-Being Scale (QWBS)
## QWBS–Self Administered (QWBS-SA)

## BRIEF DEFINITION

The **Quality of Well-Being Scale (QWBS)** was developed as part of a general health-policy model as an alternative to economic cost-benefit analysis for resource allocation. The QWBS provides a single summary score and may be used in general populations or applied to any type of condition. The QWBS score ranges from 0.0 (death) to 1.0 (asymptomatic full function).

## EXPLANATION

The QWBS assesses health-related quality of life (HRQOL) using three concepts representing related but distinct aspects of daily functioning: mobility (three levels or steps), physical activity (three steps), and social activity (five steps). A fourth concept consists of symptom/problem complexes assessing health problems or symptomatic complaints that may hinder function and well-being. The current version of the QWBS includes 26 symptom/problem complexes, whereas the new developmental self-administered version, the **QWBS–Self-Administered (QWBS–SA)**, includes 58 symptoms. Using the empirically derived general population preference values, the functioning levels are integrated with the most undesirable of the reported symptoms/problems to produce a single score or index that represents an individual's point-in-time status.

Because of the nature of the construction of the QWBS's measurement properties, internal consistency reliability is not appropriate. A study of test–retest reliability of both QWBS and QWBS-SA demonstrated the scores to be stable over a one-month time period. The reliability of day-to-day assessment indicated the interday correlations to be high (r = 0.90 or above) in populations of burn patients, chronic obstructive pulmonary disease patients, and diabetes patients.

A significant amount of data is available to support the QWBS's validity. The QWBS has been used in applied research to measure HRQOL in various disease states. Hypothesizing that QWBS scores have assessed construct validity and a number of chronic conditions should be inversely related, resulting in a Pearson correlation coefficient of −0.96.

Studies have demonstrated that the QWBS is responsive to change resulting from treatment interventions for a number of conditions. Clinical measures, pain measures, and global impression measures have been found to correlate with the QWBS.

## VALUE AND USE

The QWBS may be used in clinical trials and in evaluating screening programs for a wide range of diseases and disabilities. The QWBS may provide finer distinctions between health states than indicators, such as symptoms, chronic illnesses, and physician visits. The QWBS offers a means of complete evaluation of a health care program to estimate prognosis and operationalize "wellness."

## ISSUES

The QWBS has been criticized for being too long and complex. QWBS administration requires a trained interviewer because it involves branching and probe questions. Completion time for the interview has been reported to range from 10 to 30 minutes. Unlike the interview-based QWBS, the QWBS-SA can be self-administered in 10–15 minutes. If additional testing and application of the QWBS-SA provide evidence of its equivalence to the original, the self-administered version will reduce both respondent and administrative burden and potentially be a significantly more useful instrument.

Additionally, the QWBS has been criticized for its inability to identify the cause of a change in a score and its omission of mental health symptoms.

BIBLIOGRAPHY

Andresen EM, Rothenberg BM, Kaplan RM. Performance of a self-administered mailed version of the quality of well being (QWBS-SA) questionnaire among older adults. *Med Care.* 1998;36:1349–1360.

Kaplan RM, Anderson JP. The General Health Policy Model: an integrated approach. In: Spilker B, ed. *Quality of Life and Pharmacoeconomics in Clinical Trials.* 2nd ed. Philadelphia: Lippincott-Raven Publishers; 1996.

McDowell I, Newall C. *Measuring Health: A Guide to Rating Scales and Questionnaires.* 2nd ed. New York: Oxford University Press; 1996.

# Qualitative Research
Open-Ended Question
Focus Group

## BRIEF DEFINITION

**Qualitative research** methods aim to explore the character and meaning of human phenomena and to develop new concepts and theories to explain and describe phenomena.

## EXPLANATION

Qualitative research has a different scientific and philosophical origin than quantitative research. Qualitative researchers seek illumination, understanding, and extrapolation to similar situations instead of using statistical procedures or other methods of quantification. Therefore, qualitative analysis results in a different type of knowledge, and it also uses a different terminology than does quantitative inquiry, as shown in the table.

The objective of empirically grounded and scientifically credible qualitative research is the description or understanding of a complex human phenomenon such as a situation or a behavior. In quantitative research, hypotheses based on preexisting theory are rejected or confirmed, while in qualitative research, knowledge and theory are generated from empirical data. Preexisting theories may be used in study design but should not limit the creative process necessary for the development of new concepts that support or contradict existing theories. Qualitative researchers study phenomena in their naturalistic settings.

There are a great variety of techniques in qualitative research. The most common conceptual grounds for methods used in medicine and health services

Some Differences in General Features between Qualitative and Quantitative Research Methods

| | Qualitative | Quantitative |
|---|---|---|
| Philosophical grounds | Phenomenology, hermeneutics. | Positivism |
| Research tradition | Anthropology, sociology, nursing, psychology, family medicine. | Biomedicine, physics, chemistry, mathematics, etc. |
| Aim | Identification, description, explanation. Developing theory. | Description (rates, proportions, associations). Testing hypothesis. |
| Type of study question | What is . . . ? How? In what way? Character? Meaning? | How many? How often? Composition? Cause? Effect? |
| Design features | Field or documentary style. Focuses the issue in its context. | Experimental or survey style. Isolates the issue, disregards context. |
| Sampling | Strategic selection. Sample size may change during study. | Probability sample. Fixed selection criteria, sample size, and variables. |
| Data collection | Interviews (single or focus groups) and observations. Interactive sampling process. | Objective observations and measurements. |
| Type of data | Text. (Visual imaging, sound). | Numerical, ordinal, or nominal scales. |
| Analysis | Systematic coding, categorization, and summary. Interpretation. Cyclical process. | Statistical methods. Stepwise process. |
| Presentation of results | Categories, themes, patterns described in text. | Outcomes described in numbers. |

Reprinted from International Journal of Pediatric Othorhinolaryngology, V51: 1–10, Brunne M: "Qualitative research methods in otorhinolaryngology." © 1999 Elsevier Ireland Ltd.

research are phenomenology and grounded theory (Bunne, 1999). Qualitative research by its very nature mostly uses an **open-ended question**—that is, there are no fixed answers to choose from. Other frequently encountered methods are the Delphi Panel Method (*see term:* Delphi Panel Method) and the **focus group**.

A focus group is an organized discussions with nonrandomly selected groups of individuals about their attitudes, experiences, and perspectives on a topic. They have traditionally been used in market research but are increasingly being employed in health services research and social research. However, they should not be used as the only source of data.

VALUE AND USE

Historically qualitative research has been used in fields such as anthropology, sociology, and evaluation research. Lately the use of qualitative research methods in health services research is increasing. Qualitative research data can contribute to closing the gap between the sciences of discovery and the sciences of implementation.

In the field of health services research, qualitative methods have been used to describe many kinds of complex settings and complex interactions. These include interactions among patients, families, and clinicians. Qualitative research has its strength in the study of complex real life questions, which quantitative research (e.g., clinical trials) cannot address. For example, qualitative research methods are well suited to analyze why health education messages on stopping smoking can be well known to teenagers but not perceived as relevant to their everyday lives. Qualitative research also can find out why the results from evidence-based medicine are often not implemented in clinical practice.

Qualitative methods can also be used to generate hypotheses for subsequent quantitative research and for measurement development. The most common methods in this field are focus groups and cognitive interviews. Cognitive interviews are often considered to be an essential element of testing reliability and validity of survey instruments.

## Issues

Even though more and more researchers are using qualitative methods in the field of health services research, qualitative research has struggled to find its present position. The difference in terminology and scientific origin to positivistic tradition leads to confusion and semantic problems on the epistemological level—that is, when discussing the different kinds of knowledge and science theoretically. Some researchers emphasize a dichotomy or incompatibility of the traditional quantitative and the alternative qualitative approach due to these different theoretical foundations. However, it would be more fruitful for the relation between qualitative and quantitative methods to be characterized as complementary rather than exclusive approaches. While qualitative and quantitative research may address similar topics, each deals with a different type of question and each gets a different type of answer. Therefore both approaches should have their justification as research methods.

Qualitative research is not meant to replace quantitative research, but it is a fruitful alternative to the limits of the traditional approach.

## Bibliography

Bunne M. Qualitative research methods in otorhinolaryngology. *Int J Ped Otolraryngology.* 1999;51:1–10.

Devers KJ, Sofaer S, Rundall TG, et al. Qualitative methods in health services research—A special supplement to HSR. *Health Serv Res.* 1999;34:1101–1263.

Pope C, Mays N. Qualitative research: Reaching the parts other methods cannot reach: an introduction to qualitative research methods in health and health service research. *BMJ.* 1995;31:42–45.

Powell RA, Single HM. Focus groups. *Int J Qual Health Care.* 1996;8:499–504.

# Quantitative Research
Experimental Quantitative Research
Descriptive Quantitative Research

## BRIEF DEFINITION
**Quantitative research** is an objective, systematic process in which numerical data are analyzed with reliable statistical methods to obtain information. It is essentially objective, deductive, evaluative, and numerical. The main purpose of quantitative research is to quantify relationships between variables.

## EXPLANATION
An objective of quantitative research is to provide an independent, unbiased analysis. In gaining, analyzing, and interpreting quantitative data, the researcher attempts to remain fully detached and objective.

A second objective is to provide results that can be generalized. That is, the data are gathered in such a way that the results can be considered representative of a larger group or perhaps of the total population. For example, quantitative research attempts to reliably determine whether one drug, treatment, concept, product, package, etc., is better than the alternatives. The results from one or more quantitative studies may be projected to the population. That is, the ratio of participants in the research study reacting or answering a certain way is similar to the ratio of the total population that would have responded that way if the entire population could have been included in the study.

Quantitative research is often used to test a theory. In other words, it is a logical, deductive process of obtaining and analyzing data.

Finally, the most obvious feature of quantitative research is that the data are structured in the form of numbers or the data can be immediately converted into numbers.

## VALUE AND USE
Quantitative research is typically used to test a hypothesis. The aim is to determine the relationship between one thing (an independent variable) and another (a dependent or outcome variable) in a population. Variables are things researchers measure on subjects, which can include humans, animals, or cells. Variables can be anything that one wishes to measure, such as age, sex, weight, disease status, adverse events, health outcomes, etc.

There are two basic types of quantitative research—experimental and descriptive. Basically, **experimental quantitative research** studies are designed to examine the relationship between cause and effect (e.g., clinical drug trials). The subjects are usually measured before and after a treatment. **Descriptive quantitative research** studies examine associations between variables and do not include researcher-imposed treatments (e.g., surveys). The subjects are usually measured only once.

ISSUES

There is no universal standard for categorizing quantitative research designs. As a result, the literature contains many different names for different types of quantitative research, and many published studies do not even attempt to identify the design used. This lack of standardization may cause problems when critiquing and analyzing research.

Data obtained from quantitative research may be biased or not generalizable if the sample is not properly selected and appropriate for the study.

BIBLIOGRAPHY

Beauchamp T, Childress JF. *Principles of Biomedical Ethics.* 4th ed. New York: Oxford University Press; 1994.

Burns N, Groves SK. *The Practice of Nursing Research: Conduct, Critique & Utilization.* Philadelphia: W.B. Saunders; 1993.

Hopkins WG. Quantitative research design. *Sportscience.* 2000;4:1–8.

# Rationing

## BRIEF DEFINITION
**Rationing** is the denying or restricting of clinical services because those services, although believed to be beneficial, are too costly to provide.

## EXPLANATION
Historically the term "rationing" had a neutral or positive implication. Rationing meant distributing a scarce good fairly or equitably. Rationing when applied to health care typically carries a negative connotation in that it has come to mean withholding useful services not necessarily because they are scarce but because they are expensive.

Rationing can be explicit or covert, as when health care is controlled by a fixed budget. It is implicit or covert when care is limited through strategies such as having long waiting lists or not covering certain elective surgeries. Either way, rationing prevents people from receiving potentially beneficial services. Rationing activities have also been called health care allocation, triage, and prioritization. All refer to controlling access to health care resources when either the product/service or the financing is limited.

As different forms of rationing are imposed on health care services throughout the world, researchers struggle to define the term. Ubel and Goold (1998) point out that rationing definitions can differ in at least three ways. The first is whether the rationing is explicit (e.g., a regulation made by administrators) or whether it involves implicit mechanisms such as those created by the free market system. The second is whether rationing should be limited to cases of scarcity such as transplantable organs or whether the concept should apply to situations in which the resource is scarce only because the payer's structure controls access to certain services (e.g., referrals to specialists or prior authorization in some managed care organizations). The third is whether rationing involves only medical services necessary for survival, such as kidney dialysis, or whether it should be expanded to include all beneficial services. Ubel and Goold suggest "implicitly or explicitly allowing people to go without beneficial health care services," contending this definition provides a useful starting point for health care policy and priority-setting discussions.

All countries and medical systems ration medical care, although there are large differences in the type of criteria upon which rationing is based:

- Managed care. Managed care organizations (MCOs) in the United States have traditionally controlled costs through a variety of implicit and explicit controls including utilization review, prior authorizations, limited physician choice, restricting certain types of elective surgery, using primary care physicians as gatekeepers, and limiting drugs through a formulary and restricted drug benefit plan. Despite the widespread use of these unpopular strategies, MCOs are finding it increasingly difficult to hold down costs.

- The Oregon Health Plan (OHP). The OHP is the first public insurance plan to explicitly ration medical care and deny coverage for some health care services. It has received international attention. The OHP increased the numbers of individuals covered by Medicaid while at the same time it strictly rationed which services would be covered. In a recent evaluation of the OHP, researchers delineated reasons why it has not achieved its goals. The authors conclude that "the more that rationing decisions are made public and explicit, the less likely that a public insurance system is able to ration services" (Oberlander et al 2001).

- New Zealand. A variety of guidelines for coverage of medical care have been developed including one to ration access to end-stage renal failure programs. There is no privately funded dialysis service in New Zealand even for those willing to pay. In an analysis of the program, which they consider to be a qualified success, Feek and colleagues state, "Explicit rationing will work only when clinicians accept the link between clinical decision making and resource allocation" (Feek et al 1999).

## VALUE AND USE

Given continuing increases in health care spending, there is growing agreement on the need to control costs. A public discussion of rationing would help address actual and perceived inequalities in the delivery of health care resources.

## ISSUES

In many places including Western Europe, Canada, Australia, and New Zealand, explicit rationing systems are developed and controlled by the national and/or provincial government. In the United States, medical care is restricted primarily by private health insurers such as managed care and public agencies including Medicare and Medicaid. These programs control spending through both explicit and implicit rationing strategies. Asch and Ubel (1997) point out that disguised but pervasive rationing also occurs at the individual physician level through a variety of commonplace behaviors, including

- Thinking beyond the individual patient,
- Appealing to the "standard of care,"
- Displacing responsibility,
- Making do with less than the best, and
- Using the "best treatment" only after others fail.

Asch and Ubel point out that these situations exemplify the frequent trade-offs between cost and quality faced by physicians, patients, and insurers. They argue that "the debate should not be about some global notion of rationing or compromise, but about which justifications are valid and which compromises are appropriate."

As Mechanic (1995) states, medical care has always been rationed by available supply, distribution, and the public's ability to pay. With the increase over the past two decades in the portion of the gross national product devoted to medical care, the issue of rationing has become more important. The question is not whether there should be rationing but upon what criteria it should be based.

Frequently, there has been implicit rationing on the basis of age and/or socioeconomic status. Some of the strongest criticism against rationing has been raised against age-based rationing, which although never official, was common in Britain from the mid-1950s through the 1980s (Callahan 1996). In the United States, as the elderly population increases and the Medicare budget is stretched thinner, it appears it will be increasingly difficult to avoid some form of age-based rationing, such as the direct denial of some Medicare benefits or sharp increases in deductibles and copayments (Callahan 1996).

Evidence-based medicine and its attendant practice guidelines are sometimes advocated as the fairest approach. It has been suggested that clinical guidelines, although not usually considered rationing tools, can meet the necessary criteria of transparency (the rationale behind decisions is stated explicitly), accessibility (the criteria for inclusion and exclusion are stated in a form understandable to physicians and patients alike), justification (the exclusion criteria are justified with respect to medical and economic considerations) and universal validity (reasons for exclusion are stated in a way that is recognized as valid, impartial, and relevant) (Norheim 1999).

## BIBLIOGRAPHY

Asch DA, Ubel PA. Rationing by any other name. *N Engl J Med.* 1997;23:1668–1671.

Callahan D. Controlling the costs of health care for the elderly—fair means and foul. *N Engl J Med.* 1996;225:743–746.

Feek CM, McKean, W, Henneveld, et al. Experience with rationing health care in New Zealand. *BMJ.* 1999;318:1346–1348.

Mechanic D. Dilemmas in rationing health care services: the case for implicit rationing. *BMJ.* 1995;310:1655–1659.

Norheim OF. Healthcare rationing—are additional criteria needed for assessing evidence based clinical practice guidelines? *BMJ.* 1999;319:1426–1429.

Oberlander J, Marmoor T, Jacobs L. Rationing medical care: rhetoric and reality in the Oregon Health Plan. *CMAJ.* 2001;164:1583–1587.

Ubel PA. *Pricing Life: Why It's Time for Health Care Rationing.* Cambridge, Mass: MIT Press; 2000.

Ubel PA, Goold SD. Rationing healthcare: Not all definitions are created equal. *Arch Intern Med.* 1998;158:209–214.

# Reimbursement
Allowable Cost
Copayment
Coinsurance
Reimbursement Per Episode of Illness
Per Diem Reimbursement

## BRIEF DEFINITION
**Reimbursement** relates to public or private insurers' payment to providers for the delivery of health care products and services.

## EXPLANATION
Reimbursement rates are generally determined through negotiation with the providers of health care products or services or may be unilaterally set by the payer, who determines a reasonable price for the service (allowable cost). The **allowable cost** is the price that the provider agrees to accept as reimbursement (payment) for a specific product or service. The allowable cost can be determined by comparisons to other similar available products or services delivered by other providers, or it may be determined based on available funds in a budget. Payment of the allowable cost generally allows for better planning and management of health care resources.

Reimbursement for some products or services may not represent the entire payment to providers. The patient may be required to share a portion of the cost for a product or service either by **copayment** (a fixed payment) or **coinsurance** (a percentage of the product or services cost). For example, reimbursement to pharmacists for dispensing medications may involve a patient copayment for a portion of the cost not covered by the insurer. Copayment and coinsurance costs range and may depend upon several variables such as the $x$, the product's status on a formulary, the age of the insured, and the severity of the condition. In this example, reimbursement for the service is therefore a sum of the various forms of payment from the patient and the payer/insurer.

**Reimbursement per episode of illness** refers to reimbursement in which providers are reimbursed one sum for all services provided during the course of a specific illness, as prospectively defined. An episode includes all health care treatment and expenditures (costs) surrounding a patient care incident, such as hospitalization or an outpatient treatment. Per diem or **per diem reimbursement** is reimbursement in which providers, such as a hospital, are paid a daily rate for all services they provide. The per diem or daily rate is in lieu of reimbursement of all charges as billed by a provider in a typical fee-for-service environment. Per diems may be established for major categories of care (mental health, oncology, critical care, emergency care) and may include incremental sliding scale volume rates, ancillary services used, and mix of days by type of care used, or they may use a prospective per diem method such as average length of stay.

## Value and Use

Eligibility for reimbursement and the level of reimbursement are critical to the adoption by providers of the product, and they affect the use of the product and the commercial viability of the product or service.

In pharmacoeconomic analyses, determining an accurate payment for services is a critical component in overall or segment assessment of costs and outcomes.

## Issues

General issues to consider for use of reimbursement terminology include

- Clear identification of the patient care setting or where service is delivered,
- The date the per diem rate was set or used in addition to the time(s) of patient care service,
- Identified units of care defined in the per diem rate,
- Included or excluded cost in the per diem rate,
- Identification of the period of time or parameters surrounding the episode of illness captured in the per diem rate used for analysis, and
- The currency and exchange rate, if any, used for analysis.

## Bibliography

Centers for Medicare & Medicaid Services. http://www.cms.gov/statistics/more_statistics.asp. Accessed May 8, 2001.

Kongstvedt PR. *Essentials of Managed Health Care.* 2nd ed. Gaithersburg, Md: Aspen Publishing; 1997.

Vogenberg FR. *Introduction to Applied Pharmacoeconomics.* New York: McGraw Hill Publishing; 2001.

# Reliability
**Interrater Reliability**
**Test–Retest Reliability**
**Internal Consistency**

## Brief Definition

**Reliability** refers to the extent to which an instrument, a scale, or another type of measurement yields consistent and reproducible results. Reliability is context-specific rather than a property of an instrument under all conditions.

## Explanation

According to classical test theory, reliability of an observed score is composed of true (systematic) variance and random error. Random error represents the imprecision or noises in the observed score. The concept is used in two different types of scale validation: as a term to describe repeatability and reproducibility of measurements and as a term to evaluate multi-item scales where all items should be consistent and measure the same underlying construct (internal consistency). There are several methods of assessing reliability, each reflecting somewhat different ways of estimating random error.

*Evaluation of Repeatability Reliability*

**Interrater reliability** reflects the level of agreement between two or more raters, observers, or interviewers assessing the same target (patient or other stimuli). A high correlation indicates that the score assigned to an individual is relatively independent of who performed the rating, observation, or interview.

**Test–retest reliability** assesses the relationship of scores obtained by the same person at two or more points in time. The time period selected should be sufficiently short that the attribute of interest does not change, but long enough that respondents do not remember responses from the first assessment.

*Evaluation of Internal Consistency*

**Internal consistency** assesses the extent to which items in a scale measure a single concept and is based on item-to-item correlations in multi-item scales. It is closely related to convergent validity. Internal consistency is most frequently assessed using Cronbach's alpha. The size of coefficient alpha reflects the average correlation among items and the number of items in the scale. For parallel and some related instruments, Cronbach's alpha is an estimate of reliability.

Value and Use

Establishing the reliability of an instrument is important for several reasons:

- Reliability is a necessary but not sufficient condition for establishing validity (whether an instrument actually reflects the concept that it is intended to measure).
- Low reliability can result in a decreased probability of observing differences between groups when such differences exist.
- Knowledge of psychometric properties of an instrument in the intended context allows better selection of instruments for inclusion in a study and interpretation of study findings.

Issues

There are several issues that should be considered in the assessment of reliability. First, it must be recognized that psychometric properties of an instrument, including reliability, are context specific; that is, an instrument may exhibit adequate reliability in one situation or with one subgroup, but not another. Reliability must always be assessed in the target population. Second, it is important to consider the question being asked when selecting and interpreting instrument reliability. Some types of reliability are appropriate for a specific situation and others are not. For example, interrater reliability is important when an instrument is interviewer-administered, but less so when the mode of administration is self-report unless proxy and patient responses will be mixed. In a longitudinal study, test–retest reliability is important, but internal consistency of the scale may or may not be important. Third, interpretation of the size of a reliability coefficient depends on how the instrument will be used. All other things being equal, higher coefficients are better. However, a very high alpha coefficient may indicate undesirable redundancy in the scale, and lower reliability coefficients may be acceptable in studies with larger sample sizes. Guidelines for interpreting reliability coefficients are available (Nunnally & Bernstein 1994; Hays et al 1998).

Traditionally, health researchers have relied on reliability coefficients based on classical test theory as described above. However, newer methods of reliability assessment should also be considered when conducting a reliability assessment. Three methods increasingly seen in the literature include generalizability theory, factor analysis, and item response theory (Cronbach et al 1963, Hambleton et al 1991, Nunnally & Bernstein 1994).

BIBLIOGRAPHY

Cronbach LJ, Gleser GC, Rajaratnam N. Theory of generalizability: a liberalization of reliability theory. *Brit J Math Stat Psychol.* 1963;16:137–173.

Hambleton RK, Swaminathan H, Rogers L. *Fundamentals of Item Response Theory.* Newbury Park, Calif: Sage, 1991.

Hays RD, Anderson RT, Revicki D. Assessing reliability and validity of measurement in clinical trials. In: Staquet MJ, Hays RD, Fayers PM, eds. *Quality of Life Assessment in Clinical Trials: Methods and Practice.* New York: Oxford University Press; 1998.

Nunnally JC, Bernstein IH. *Psychometric Theory.* 3rd ed. New York: McGraw-Hill; 1994.

Patrick DL, Erickson P. *Health Status and Health Policy: Allocating Resources to Health Care.* New York: Oxford University Press; 1993.

# Research Entities

Sponsor
Funding Agency
Contracting Agency
Contract Research Organization (CRO)
Site
Practice Research Network
Trials Management Organization (TMO)

Principal Investigator
Coinvestigator
Coordinating Center
Steering Committee
Human Subjects Committee
Ethics Committee

BRIEF DEFINITION

**Research entities** are organizations or individuals involved in soliciting, planning, funding, conducting, and evaluating research. Depending on the nature of the research and its funding, different entities may be involved in any portion of a particular research project.

EXPLANATION

The research process can be complex with a large number of entities involved. The specifics vary based on the project and the nature of the funding, structure of the study, and the organizations involved.

Funding can be provided from a variety of sources. The most common funding entities are government agencies, private foundations, and equipment or pharmaceutical manufacturers. The funding entity is frequently called the **sponsor** of the research, although this term is most commonly applied when the funding entity is a manufacturer or a private foundation. If funding comes from government or nonprofit sources, the term "sponsor" is less commonly used. Commonly used terms for federally funded research include **funding agency** or **contracting agency** (if the funding is based on a contract).

Research can be performed by a variety of organizations, including an academic institution (university and hospital), private consulting firm or corporation, pharmaceutical manufacturer, and a **contract research organization (CRO)**. A CRO is a corporate entity that specializes in facilitating the conduct of clinical research on behalf of, and on a contractual basis with, corporate and governmental sponsors. The CRO may engage in all aspects of study design, implementation, and analysis, or it may be contracted to provide only some of these services.

Many clinical trials are performed at multiple locations or sites. A **site** is a clinical setting where the trial investigators are located, the patients are receiving their care, and the technology being evaluated is delivered. Sites can include academic medical centers, nonacademic community hospitals, group practices, individual physician offices, and managed care organizations. Some research is performed using a **practice research network**. A practice research network is an organization of physicians and practices that solicit or create research studies that are then performed by the network members at their individual practice sites. Some multi-center trials may use the services of a **trials management organization (TMO)** or site management organization (SMO). This organization is a corporate entity that assists in implementing clinical trials by facilitating investigator selection and recruitment and relationships between the sponsor, the CRO, and individual trial sites.

The lead researcher in a study is called the **principal investigator**. For multi-center clinical trials, a participating researcher is frequently called a **coinvestigator**. The administration of large multi-center trials is frequently organized into different functional entities. Data collection and analysis may be assigned to the **coordinating center**. A sponsor may also convene a **steering committee** comprising the principal investigator, coinvestigators, and other additional experts to oversee a multi-center study. Other functional entities may include a monitoring entities in clinical trials or data and safety monitoring board (DSMB) (*see term:* Monitoring Entity – Clinical Trials), which is composed of researchers, ideally independent of the trials they monitor, who periodically review data from blinded trials. A DSMB can stop a trial early if treatment-related harms are detected or if treatment is proven beneficial. An independent data-monitoring committee (IDMC) performs a similar function for a study's sponsor and can recommend terminating or modifying a study based on results to date.

To protect the rights of study subjects, review by an independent entity is required. The exact structure, titles, and duties of these oversight committees vary from institution to institution. Titles include institutional review board (IRB), **human subjects committee**, and **ethics committee**. Institutional review board (IRB) is the most commonly used term and generally refers to an administrative panel at a clinical site that approves the conduct of all trials or other studies (within the site) that involve data collection from human subjects (at that site). "IRB approval" of the study protocol, consent forms, and data collection forms is typically required for each site included in the research project. Some institutions have a human subjects committee that specifically looks at issues relating to human subjects while the IRB looks at the overall study quality and ethics. In some institutions a separate ethics committee may also look at the ethical implications of a study.

## Responsiveness
Distribution-Based Method
Anchor-Based Method
Minimal Clinical Importance Difference (MCID)

BRIEF DEFINITION

The **responsiveness** of an instrument relates to the instrument's ability to detect clinically meaningful changes over time when a patient improves or deteriorates.

EXPLANATION

An evaluative instrument requires good responsiveness. The term "instrument responsiveness" relates to the ability of an instrument to detect changes within patients. The term "instrument sensitivity," on the other hand, relates to the ability of an instrument to detect differences between groups—for example, between two treatment groups in a randomized controlled trial, or between groups of patients with mild disease and severe disease. While the same type of methodology can apply to both responsiveness and sensitivity, this section focuses on within-patient change—that is, responsiveness. When there is a change in the health state of an individual, an instrument should be able to detect that change even if it is small. There are two common approaches to determining clinically meaningful differences:

A **distribution-based method** focuses on a signal-to-noise ratio, specifically a ratio of a difference in means to the variability in scores. Distribution-based approaches tend to share the same numerator. For within-group change, the numerator tends to be the difference between the mean score at follow-up minus the mean score at baseline in a group of patients. What tends to differ is the estimate of variability in the denominator. Measures of responsiveness include the effect size, with standard deviation of baseline scores in the denominator; standardized responsiveness mean, with the standard deviation of change scores in the denominator; responsive statistic, with the standard deviation of change scores in patients who remain stable in the denominator; paired t-statistic, with the standard error of change scores in the denominator; and the standardized error of measurement, which is a function of the baseline standard deviation and the reliability coefficient of the instrument.

An **anchor-based method** examines the relationship between scores on an instrument whose interpretation is under question (the target instrument) and some external standard (the anchor). Anchor-based approaches may vary because there are potentially multiple anchors. For example, prospectively measured change in an instrument can be compared with a change in a clinical parameter (e.g., viral load) or with a retrospective report of global change (e.g., much better, a little better, about the same, a little worse, much worse). Whether a single anchor or multiple anchors are used, anchors must be interpretable and exhibit an appreciable association with the target instrument.

VALUE AND USE

A crucial task for patients and health care professionals concerns the interpretation of results from an instrument on measuring and evaluating observed changes. Is the observed change clinically important—that is, does it exceed minimally important difference to the patient and other stakeholders? Or should it be considered trivial or insufficient to support treatment? An instrument may be of limited applicability if it is not responsive to individual changes over time. Responsiveness can also be regarded as providing additional evidence of validity of an instrument when it confirms that the anticipated responses occur when the patient's status changes. An instrument may be deemed responsive, for example, when the mean changes in its scores correspond, as expected, to categories of an anchor on patients' global rating of change. Measures of responsiveness can be applied and interpreted on a relative basis, instead of an absolute one, to compare different scales (domains) of the same instrument or to compare different instruments in order to determine which one is most responsive. For instance, among several generic instruments, one in particular may be deemed the most responsive based on the effect size and standard response mean in a specific study population.

ISSUES

Responsiveness has also been viewed as the ability of a particular instrument in a specific application to detect the **minimal clinical importance difference (MCID)**, the smallest difference in a score that is considered worthwhile or important. As descriptors of change, distribution-based and anchor-based measures of instrument responsiveness do not by themselves indicate whether the change is minimally important to the decision maker. But they are often interpreted and used in order to arrive at an absolute minimum number that must be exceeded before a difference is worth considering. Several issues emanate from this.

First, such an absolute threshold might be suspect because it ignores the cost of resources to produce a change. Second, the estimated magnitude varies as it depends on the distributional index or the external standard used. Third, the amount of change might depend on the direction of change (improvement versus worsening). Fourth, the meaning of change might depend on initial health status. Fifth, uncertainty may arise about whether lack of observed change reflects true absence of change or whether the research design and analysis may have obscured meaningful change. Sixth, distribution-based methods might not suffice on their own but might be useful to the extent that they bear a consistent relationship with anchor-based methods. Finally, even anchor-based methods might require validation with alternative anchors.

### BIBLIOGRAPHY

Fayers PM, Machin D. *Quality of Life: Assessment, Analysis, and Interpretation.* West Sussex, England: John Wiley & Sons Ltd; 2000.

Hays RD, Woolley JM. The concept of clinically meaningful difference in health-related quality-of-life research. *Pharmacoeconomics.* 2000;18:419–423.

Kazis LE, Anderson JJ, Meenan RF. Effect sizes for interpreting changes in health status. *Medical Care.* 1989;(suppl) 27:S178–S189.

# Retrospective Analysis

### BRIEF DEFINITION

**Retrospective analysis** is an analysis based on currently available data, generally from administrative data systems such as medical claims, managed care encounter data, hospital discharge data, or electronic medical records (*see term:* Epidemiology).

### EXPLANATION

Retrospective database studies examine the health care utilization of patients in real-world settings. They can focus on either economic or clinical outcomes and can be conducted from a variety of perspectives including those of patients, health care providers, payers, and society. In fact, the defining characteristic of retrospective studies is that they involve the analysis of data that has already been collected—usually for some purpose other than the study at hand.

### VALUE AND USE

Retrospective analyses are valuable because they provide information about health care treatments in real-world settings. Retrospective databases are often very large (sometimes containing information on millions of individuals) and, because the information has already been collected, retrospective studies can be carried out more quickly than clinical trials or prospective observational studies.

### ISSUES

The main advantage of retrospective analysis—that they are based on large samples of patient populations in real world settings—is also their main disadvantage. The databases used for retrospective analysis are not usually designed with research in mind. As a result, data quality may be poor (e.g., incomplete coding of diagnoses or procedures, discontinuous enrollment of patients), important clinical data may be lacking (e.g., lab test results, clinical measures of disease severity), and a variety of statistical problems (e.g., sample selection bias) may threaten the validity of conclusions based upon retrospective analysis. Also, the results of retrospective studies may be invalid due to changes in clinical practice and/or reimbursement after data was collected.

BIBLIOGRAPHY

Anderson, C. Measuring what works in health care. *Science.* 1994;268:1080–1082.
Arnold R, Kotsanos J, Motheral B, et al. Panel 3: Methodological issues in conducting pharmacoeconomic evaluations—retrospective and claims database studies. *Value Health.* 1999;2:82–87.
Garnick D, Hendricks A, Comstock C. Measuring quality of care: Fundamental information from administrative datasets. *Int J Qual Health Care.* 1994;6:163–177.
McGlynn EA, Damberg CL, Kerr EA, Brook RH. *Health Information Systems Designs Issues and Analytic Applications.* Santa Monica, Calif: Rand Health; 1998.
Motheral B, Brooks J, Clark MA, et al. A checklist for retrospective database studies—report of the ISPOR task force on retrospective databases. *Value Health.* 2003;6:90–97.

# Risk

**Attributable Risk**
**Population Attributable Risk**
**Relative Risk**

BRIEF DEFINITION

**Risk** refers to the proportion of the population who, on average, will contract the disease of interest over a specified period of time (*see term:* Epidemiology).

EXPLANATION

In order to determine risk, one must first define the time period to be studied, or "risk period." Once a time period is stated, risk can be calculated by the following equation:

$$\text{Risk} = \frac{\text{Newly Affected Persons}}{\text{Total Persons Observed}} \times 100 \text{ (for percentage)}$$

This is known as the "crude rate" of disease, as it is merely the number of new cases relative to the entire population. Crude rates can often be misinterpreted due to nonspecified, underlying causes, such as growth of certain categories of the population. In order to account for these possible differences, "standardized rates" are created. These rates are statistically constructed summary rates that account for the population differences with respect to the variables (categories) themselves. In order to directly standardize the rates, for instance to compare two populations, the rates of incidence must be compared to a standard population.

VALUE AND USE

Risk can be used to indicate the probability of developing disease for an individual or a given population over a specific time period. It is often used to study or monitor the occurrence of disease in populations.

ISSUES

The flu vaccine is a good example of the use of risk measurement. With the many different strains of flu virus known, it would be difficult, if not impossible, to vaccinate a population for every virus. Risk is calculated and used to determine the three most likely strains to be contracted for a season, and the vaccine is created for those specific strains. Knowing the risk makes the flu vaccination program much more economical.

BIBLIOGRAPHY

Greenberg RS, Daniels SR, Flanders WD, et al. *Medical Epidemiology.* Stamford, Conn: Appleton and Lange; 1996.
Hennekens CH, Buring JE. *Epidemiology in Medicine.* Boston: Little, Brown and Company; 1987.

## Attributable Risk

BRIEF DEFINITION

**Attributable risk** is a measure used to explain the excess of disease in exposed individuals versus those who are unexposed.

EXPLANATION

Also known as the "risk difference," this measurement indicates the percentage of disease associated completely with exposure to the disease. Instead of dividing the percentage diseased of exposed individuals by the percentage diseased of unexposed individuals, as in relative risk, attributable risk is calculated by subtracting the unexposed, as in the following equation:

Attributable Risk (Risk Difference) =

$$\frac{\text{Diseased Exposed Individuals} - \text{Diseased Unexposed Individuals}}{\text{Total Exposed Individuals} - \text{Total Unexposed Individuals}}$$

By removing the disease that "would have happened anyway" from the disease of those exposed, the end result is the disease "attributable" to the exposure.

VALUE AND USE

Attributable risk is used to measure how much of the risk in exposed persons would be prevented if the exposure were eliminated.

ISSUES

Perhaps one of the most famous instances of the use of attributable risk was in the beginning epidemiology of AIDS. The use of this measurement aided investigators in determining a link between homosexuality and the symptoms associated with AIDS.

BIBLIOGRAPHY

Hennekens CH, Buring JE. *Epidemiology in Medicine.* Boston: Little, Brown and Company; 1987.

## Population Attributable Risk

BRIEF DEFINITION

**Population attributable risk** is a measure of the excess rate of disease in the total study population of exposed and unexposed individuals that is attributable to the exposure.

EXPLANATION

Also known as the "population attributable rate," this measurement makes attributable risk more applicable to the entire population by including total population data in the estimation. There are two primary methods of determining population attributable risk:

$$\text{Population Attributable Risk} = \frac{\text{Total Exposed Individuals}}{\text{Attributable Risk} \times \text{Total Individuals}}$$

This first method assumes previous calculation of attributable risk and adjusts to determine the rate of disease due to exposure for the entire population.

$$\text{Population Attributable Risk} = \frac{\text{Diseased Individuals} - \text{Diseased Unexposed Individuals}}{\text{Total Individuals} - \text{Total Unexposed Individuals}}$$

This second method results in the same estimate, but better shows how the population attributable risk is merely the percent of total disease minus the disease that "would have happened anyway."

VALUE AND USE

Population attributable risk has important public health implications. It is used to measure how much of the risk in the total population (including both exposed and unexposed persons) would be prevented if the exposure were eliminated.

ISSUES
When determining the risk for myocardial infarctions in Americans, it is not enough to measure the attributable risk in a certain group of the population, such as middle-aged Caucasian males. In addition to this, one must apply this risk to the population, so that other groups of the population are taken into consideration.

BIBLIOGRAPHY
Hennekens CH, Buring JE. *Epidemiology in Medicine.* Boston: Little, Brown and Company; 1987.

## Relative Risk

BRIEF DEFINITION
**Relative risk** is a measure used to predict the likelihood of disease in exposed individuals relative to those who are unexposed.

EXPLANATION
Also known as "risk ratio," this measurement indicates the number of times more likely an individual is to contract a disease when exposed versus unexposed. For instance, people who cut themselves on a rusty nail might be "5.4" times more likely to contract tetanus than people who do not cut themselves. The "5.4" is the relative risk measurement and can be determined by the following equation:

Relative Risk (Risk Ratio)  =

$$\frac{\text{Diseased Exposed Individuals} \div \text{Total Exposed Individuals}}{\text{Diseased Unexposed Individuals} \div \text{Total Unexposed Individuals}}$$

By calculating the proportion of exposed individuals who contracted the disease and dividing by the percentage of unexposed individuals who contracted disease, you can determine the factor of likelihood that one will contract the disease relative to his or her exposure status.

VALUE AND USE
Relative risk is used to measure the strength of the association between disease and exposure. If there is no association, the relative risk would be equal to 1. If the exposure increases the risk of disease, the relative risk would be greater than 1. Otherwise, the relative risk would be less than 1.

ISSUES
Relative risk can be used in many different contexts, not just disease. Relative risk is calculated to help determine which vehicles are "more likely" to roll over in an accident. This measurement tells how strong a risk factor the measured variable is.

BIBLIOGRAPHY

Hennekens CH, Buring JE. *Epidemiology in Medicine.* Boston: Little, Brown and Company; 1987.

# Risk Adjustment

BRIEF DEFINITION

**Risk adjustment** is a method of accounting for the morbidity of individual patients when making aggregate comparisons between population outcomes (*see terms:* Epidemiology, Risk).

EXPLANATION

Since the 1970s, many studies have documented unexplained variation in outcomes between groups of "similar" patient populations. In addition, the implementation of the DRG payment system in the 1980s is based on grouping patients with "similar" conditions. The assumption is that the patient groups are similar. Valid comparison of outcomes between groups of patients requires measurement of the outcome and a method to "adjust" for individual patient risks for the outcome to make sure the groups are made up of "similar" patients. The goal of risk adjustment is to account for extraneous patient or disease characteristics prior to making comparative inferences based on outcome data. Thus, risk adjustment uses complex algorithms and models to remove or reduce the effects of a confounding factor or risk factor, when assessing outcomes. Examples of risk factors used in models include patient demographic characteristics (e.g., age and gender), principal diagnosis code (e.g., case mix), comorbid conditions (e.g., number and severity), and severity of principal diagnosis. Thus, it is important to understand that risk adjustment models use different risk factors to predict different outcomes. Risk factors in the model are tailored to predict the outcome being adjusted.

Varying types of outcomes may be adjusted for risk. Outcomes range from resource use such as cost and length of stay to mortality. Different patient risk factors may be used to adjust different outcomes for the same population. For example, the risk factors used to adjust for mortality may be different than the factors used to adjust for cost. It is intuitive that patients who enter the hospital and expire after two days may be different from the patients who have high costs. It is equally intuitive that different risk factors would predict the two different outcomes. The model to adjust mortality may not and probably should not be the same as the model to adjust cost.

Several risk adjustment models with different objectives have been developed to help policy decision makers compare groups of patients. Most models work by clustering diagnoses, patient demographic characteristics, procedure codes, admission source, and other information into clinically meaningful categories for an individual patient to give a composite measure of risk that can help predict the outcome of concern. What data is used to construct the model is controversial. Many risk models rely on administrative databases or claims data to generate model data. Thus, the population of interest is critical. Adjusting mortality for all hospitalized patients is not the same as adjusting mortality for renal transplant patients.

## VALUE AND USE

The goal of all outcomes information is to improve those outcomes and the quality of care provided to the patient. Risk adjustment plays a role in the concept of comparing outcomes between groups of patients. Patient groups may be logically defined in many ways. For example, they may be grouped by geographic location (e.g., region or hospital), clinical manifestation of disease or treatment (e.g., patients with congestive heart failure or patients who have had a recent heart valve replacement surgery), provider characteristic (e.g., physician specialty or location of the provider) and any other way of grouping patients. Comparison of patient groups is important to public policy decision makers. Risk-adjusted outcomes are used for a broad range of policy-related purposes, including provider reimbursement, provider profiling and monitoring the quality of care. Risk adjustment is used to adjust capitation payment to providers to ensure that adverse selection does not occur. In other words, risk adjustment can ensure that providers caring for patients with complex medical problems are not penalized. Risk adjustment aids in the comparison of practice patterns across providers to monitor performance. Efforts to increase accountability for the resources consumed and quality produced point to the need to make valid comparisons. Finally, risk adjustment is used to monitor the health of a population and accounts for morbidity. Traditional measures of population health such as mortality rates or any incidence rate do not tell the story of population health. Risk adjustment helps by using the traditional outcomes after adjusting for morbidity and other risk factors.

## ISSUES

One significant issue is the administrative complexity in accomplishing risk adjustment. Administrative databases (e.g., diagnosis based models) are used since that data is readily available. Clinical data is lacking and expensive to collect. Often, risk adjustment is limited to the data available and the models that have already been developed. The end result is that much of the variation in the outcome of interest remains unaccounted for even after risk adjustment. A related limitation is the accuracy of the coding of the diagnoses. Incomplete or inaccurate coding (such as "up coding") can severely impact the validity of a risk adjustment model. Finally, it is important to note that different risk adjustment models will produce different risk-adjusted results for the same outcome. This scenario occurs due to the models using different definitions of risk or risk factors. It is no surprise that controversy exists on which model is "correct."

BIBLIOGRAPHY

Iezzoni LI. *Risk Adjustment for Measuring Health Care Outcomes.* Ann Arbor, Mich: Healthcare
    Administration Press; 1997.
Iezzoni LI. The risks of risk adjustment. *JAMA.* 1997;278:1600–1607.
Kuttner R. The risk adjustment debate. *N Engl J Med.* 1998;339:1952–1956.

# Rosser Index

BRIEF DEFINITION

The **Rosser Index** is a two-dimensional classification system of health states,
developed by Rachel Rosser (1972). The Rosser Index measures health outcomes along the two dimensions of disability and distress. The index summarizes a total of 32 health states by combining eight levels of disability and four
levels of distress. (*See terms:* Health Utilities Index, Utility)

EXPLANATION

Levels of disability in the index are

1. No disability
2. Slight disability which only interferes with social life
3. Severe social disability and/or slight impairment of performance at work
4. Choice of work or performance at work severely limited. Housewives and
   old people able to do light housework only, but able to go out shopping
5. Unable to undertake any paid employment. Unable to continue education.
   Housewives only able to perform a few simple tasks. Old people confined to
   home except for escorted outings and short walks and unable to do shopping
6. Confined to a chair or a wheelchair or able to move around in the home
   only with support from an assistant
7. Confined to bed
8. Unconscious

Levels of distress in the index are

1. No distress
2. Slight distress
3. Moderate distress
4. Severe distress

VALUE AND USE

The Rosser Index has been used as a classification system for measuring health
outcomes. However, as is the case with other preference-based measures, acceptance of the underlying methodology awaits more consensus and documented

evidence of its validity, reliability, and responsiveness. The robustness and quality of the latter will determine the value for its use in economic evaluation in health care.

## ISSUES

Issues surrounding the Rosser Index include the following:

- Initial valuations of alternative combinations of disability and distress are derived from a very small sample (70).
- Both patients and their proxies have identified health states that they consider to be worse than death (being confined to bed in severe distress and being unconscious and in no distress).
- Limited evidence is available on congruence of Rosser Index values and other health state preference measures.
- It is not much used anymore. It has been superseded by more recent utility-weighted indexes.

## BIBLIOGRAPHY

Hollingworth W, Mackenzie R, Todd CJ, Dixon AK. Measuring changes in quality of life following magnetic resonance imaging of the knee: SF-36, EuroQol or Rosser index? *Qual Life Res.* 1995;4:325–334.

Rosser R, Kind P. A scale of valuations of states of illness: is there a social consensus? *Int J Epidemiol.* 1978;7;347–358.

Rosser RM, Watts VC. The measurement of hospital output. *Int J of Epidemiol.* 1972;1:361–368.

# Sample Selection Model

## BRIEF DEFINITION

A **sample selection model** is a model that tests and provides a statistical correction for the presence of sample selection bias.

## EXPLANATION

A sample selection model tests and provides a statistical correction for sample selection bias (*see term:* Clinical Trial – Study Bias). Sample selection bias refers to bias due to unobserved factors associated with treatment selection (e.g., physician prescribing preferences, patient illness severity) that are also correlated with treatment outcomes.

## VALUE AND USE

In any nonrandomized study, selection bias is a potential threat to the validity of conclusions reached. Failure to account for sample selection bias can lead to conclusions about treatment effectiveness or treatment cost that are not really due to the treatment at all, but rather to the unobserved factors that are correlated with both treatment and outcome. Sample selection models provide a test for the presence of selection bias. These models also provide a correction for selection bias, enabling an investigator to obtain unbiased estimates of treatment effects.

## ISSUES

The estimation method for controlling the effects of nonrandom sample attrition bias involves two steps. In the first step, a probit model of attrition is estimated. The estimated probabilities from the probit model, which are a function of observable variables, are then used to calculate a variable known as the inverse mills ratio. This variable is intended to measure the unobserved factors that may be correlated with treatment outcomes. The outcome equation is estimated in the second step. In the outcome equation, the estimated inverse mills ratio from the first equation is entered as an additional explanatory variable using observations. The inverse mills ratio captures the effects of unobserved variables on the outcome variable—enabling unbiased estimates to be obtained for the parameters associated with the observed variables—in particular, treatment effects.

A variety of factors influence how well sample selection models actually work in practice. For example, if the observed variables used to model the probability of attrition from the trial are exactly the same as those used to model the outcome variable in the second equation, the inverse mills ratio will tend to be highly correlated with the observed variables in the second equation. In this case, sample selection models will not provide a reliable test for the presence of sample selection bias, nor an effective control for it. On the other hand, if it is possible to identify different sets of observable variables in the models of treatment selection and outcomes (even if there is significant overlap between them), sample selection models tend to be much more effective in controlling for selection bias.

BIBLIOGRAPHY

Crown W, Obenchain R, Englehart L, et al. Application of sample selection models to outcomes research: the case of evaluating effects of antidepressant therapy on resource utilization. *Stat Med*. 1998;17:1943–1958.

D'Agostino R. Tutorial in biostatistics: Propensity score methods for bias reduction in the comparison of a treatment to a non-randomized control group. *Stat Med*. 1998;17:2265–2281.

Heckman J. The common structure of statistical models of truncation, sample selection, and limited dependent variables and a simple estimator for such models. *Annals of Economic and Social Measurement*. 1976;5:475–492.

Heckman J. Sample selection bias as a specification error. *Econometrica*. 1979;47:153–161.

Rosenbaum P, Rubin D. Reducing bias in observational studies using subclassification on the propensity score. *J Am Stat Assoc*. 1984;79:516–524.

# Sensitivity Analysis
## Tornado Diagram

### BRIEF DEFINITION

**Sensitivity analysis** is a way to analyze the impact of uncertainty on an economic analysis or a decision (*see terms:* Decision Analysis, Decision Tree, Modeling). The simplest form of sensitivity analysis is a one-way analysis—that is, changing the value of one variable through the range of plausible values while keeping the other variables constant. A **tornado diagram** is a set of one-way sensitivity analyses brought together in a single graph, with the most critical variable in terms of impact at the top of the graph and the rest ranked according to their impact thereafter; hence the term "tornado diagram," as it looks like a tornado or funnel.

### EXPLANATION

Estimates of costs, effectiveness, and cost-effectiveness that are obtained as a result of any analysis may be subject to uncertainty for any of several reasons. There may be uncertainty regarding the parameters used in the analysis—for example, due to a lack of existing data, only imprecise estimates may be available or value judgments may be needed to determine the value used. Also, while in reality the values of a parameter may be randomly distributed within a certain range, the analysis is often based on single point estimates such as the mean.

There may also be uncertainty around the model used to analyze the results— for example, uncertainty regarding how to combine the parameters or how to generalize the results.

Therefore, the impact of uncertainty should be assessed, and the most influential parameters and their impacts on the study results should be identified, quantified, and interpreted. There are several ways to deal with uncertainty, including simple ways such as one-way sensitivity analysis, two or multi-way sensitivity analysis, threshold analysis, scenario analysis and more complex approaches making use of mathematical theory, and statistics, such as Monte Carlo simulation, bootstrapping, and so on (*see terms:* Bootstrapping, Modeling).

One-way analysis represents the simplest and most commonly used approach to deal with uncertainty in health outcomes studies. In this context, the value of one variable is varied within a range of plausible values, while the other variables in the analysis are kept constant, and the single variable's impact on the main study result is quantified and examined. For example, the effect of the rate used to discount costs and health benefits in an economic evaluation can be significant in cases in which the analysis has a long-term horizon. One may choose to apply at baseline any of the different rates proposed and utilized in the literature, including 0% (i.e., not to discount), 2%, 3%, 4%, 5%, and 6%. Then, in the context of a one-way sensitivity analysis, the discounting rate can be varied from 0% to 6%, and the impact on the main study result (e.g., incremental cost per life year saved with treatment A relative to treatment B) can be studied, and some inferences on the robustness of the results can be drawn.

A tornado diagram is a series of one-way sensitivity analyses brought together in a single graph. It consists of a simple way to summarize and depict graphically the impacts of many different variables underlying an analysis on the main study result or variable of interest. First, a range of plausible values is assigned to each variable being analyzed, and the corresponding values on the main study result are recorded. A horizontal bar is then generated for each variable, where each bar reflects the values of the main study result or variable of interest upon which the sensitivity analysis is being conducted, corresponding to a range of different values of the underlying variable. A wide bar indicates that the related variable is very critical in terms of its large potential effect on the expected study result and vice versa. The widest bar is at the top and the narrowest at bottom, resulting in a funnel-like appearance. The tornado diagram also includes a dotted line, showing the original (baseline) result.

The example below shows the impact of four independent factors, such as patient age, and a decision taken by the analyst, such as the discounting rate applied, on the expected incremental cost per life year gained with treatment A relative to treatment B. Age is the most influential variable, with 45 years corresponding to an incremental cost-effectiveness ratio (ICER) of 11500 USD and 75 years of age corresponding to an ICER of 25000 USD. This is a hypothetical illustration; a real example can be found in Chancellor et al (2001).

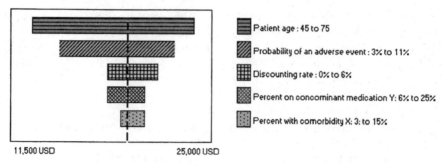

11,500 USD                    25,000 USD

Incremental cost per life year gained

Tornado Diagram: key factors influencing the ICER of treatment A versus B

## VALUE AND USE

As noted earlier, the results of health outcomes or pharmacoeconomic studies are subject to a degree of uncertainty, which needs to be assessed, especially in light of the fact that such studies are used in decision making. Sensitivity analyses and tornado diagrams represent a relatively easy and straightforward approach to interpreting the results and assessing the robustness of the results obtained from a particular analysis. Often, because of data limitations, sensitivity analysis represents the only tool available for assessing uncertainty around a set of results.

However, one-way analysis may be overly simplistic in representing reality. Although it can well represent the impact of a change in only one or two variables in a certain predetermined direction, the reality is typically more complex. In reality, many different combinations of variables may be possible, and variables may be associated with each other.

Nevertheless, tornado diagrams represent a useful graphical tool to summarize and portray the results of one-way analyses. It is important that they be updated as new studies are performed and new knowledge accumulated. As well, when additional data exist, such as individual patient data on health outcomes and resource utilization and costs collected within randomized controlled clinical trials, then more robust approaches can be used in dealing with uncertainty. Various mathematical and statistical approaches are described in Drummond et al (1997).

## ISSUES

Due to the growing importance of health outcome studies in health care decision making, it is important to ensure that uncertainty is dealt with in a robust manner. The conduct of sensitivity analysis and the presentation of results in tornado diagrams help analysts and decision makers to be explicit with respect to the key drivers of uncertainty in a model. Because sensitivity analysis involves significant analyst discretion (as the analyst chooses which variables to vary and the amount of variation), it is critical that good research practices be followed in this area to promote valid results. Briggs (1995) has produced guidelines for presenting the results of sensitivity analysis in economic evaluation, but in general few generally agreed-upon guidelines exist on how to conduct or interpret sensitivity analyses in different types of health outcomes or pharmacoeconomic or economic evaluation studies.

BIBLIOGRAPHY

Briggs AH. *Handling Uncertainty in the Results of Economic Evaluation.* OHE Briefing no. 32. London: Office of Health Economics; 1995.

Chancellor J, Hunsche E, de Cruz E, Sarasin FP. Economic evaluation of celecoxib, a new Cyclo-Oxygenase 2 specific inhibitor in Switzerland. *Pharmacoeconomics.* 2001;19:59–75.

Drummond MF, O'Brien B, Stoddart GL, et al. *Methods for the Economic Evaluation of Health Care Programmes.* London: Oxford University Press, 1997.

# Severity of Illness

## BRIEF DESCRIPTION

**Severity of illness** is a component of risk adjustment (*see terms:* Risk, Risk Adjustment). It describes the extent or state of the disease existing in patients prior to an intervention.

## EXPLANATION

Severity adjustment and risk adjustment are often used interchangeably. However, severity of illness is only one factor used for risk adjustment. Other factors such as patient sociodemographics, comorbid illness, and preferences can be equally essential for adequate risk adjustment. A widespread example of disease severity is cancer staging, which is based on the degree of growth/spread of the malignancy. While cancer stage is highly predictive of mortality risk, other factors such as comorbid illness or patient age may also explain risk.

Severity of illness measures attempt to differentiate among patients with respect to the state of their disease. For the most part, disease severity scores have been created to estimate a patient's risk of morbidity or mortality based on a number of clinical measures related to the illness itself. These scores are used in conjunction with other variables (e.g., sociodemographic factors, comorbid conditions, functional status, etc.) to provide a balanced and fair comparison in instances where there is a risk of biased results due to heterogeneous comparison groups.

## VALUE AND USE

Several disease severity scores have been created for use in the inpatient setting, such as APACHE, DS-Clin, DS-Scale, Medisgroups. These scores have generally been created using statistical methods that estimate the correlation between certain parameters and the likelihood of an event occurring, and they have been found to be highly predictive of outcomes such as mortality. Inclusion of these scores in risk adjustment models can significantly increase explanatory power versus using socioeconomic variables and/or comorbid illness alone.

## ISSUES

To date, the majority of severity measures have been focused on the inpatient setting, due to the availability of detailed clinical data, the intensity of care (and associated cost) in this setting, and the recent increase in interest in patient outcomes due to hospital accreditation. Therefore, use of these scores in conditions and patients outside the hospital setting has been of limited success. Within the hospital setting, disease severity scores have been predictive of in-hospital and 30-day mortality, but less explanatory for resource utilization or hospital length of stay.

## BIBLIOGRAPHY

Iezzoni LI. Judging hospitals by severity-adjusted mortality rates: the influence of severity adjustment method. *Am J Pub Health.* 1996;86:1379–1387.

Iezzoni LI. *Risk Adjustment for Measuring Health Care Outcomes.* Ann Arbor, Mich: Healthcare Administration Press; 1997.

Schwarz M. Do severity measures explain differences in length of hospital stay: the case of hip fracture. *Health Serv Res.* 1996;31:365–385.

Thomas JW, Longo DR. Application of severity measurement systems for hospital quality measurement. *Hosp Health Serv Admin.* 1990;35:221–243.

# Short Form 36 (SF-36)

**SF-36 Health Survey**
**RAND 36-Item Health Survey 1.0**
**Health Status Questionnaire**
**RAND-36 Health Status Inventory (HSI)**

## BRIEF DEFINITION

The **Short Form 36 (SF-36)** is a widely-used 36-item generic health status questionnaire (*see term:* Health Status, Health-Related Quality of Life).

## EXPLANATION

The Short Form 36 was developed by the Rand Corporation in the United States for use in the Health Insurance Experiment/Medical Outcomes Study (HIS/MOS). It comprises 36 items selected from a larger pool of items used by RAND in the MOS. As a generic health status profile, the SF-36 includes multiple item scales measuring the following eight health concepts: physical functioning, role limitations because of physical problems, bodily pain, social functioning, general mental health (psychological distress and psychological well-being), role limitations due to emotional problems, vitality (energy/fatigue), and general health perceptions. In addition to eight domain scores, the SF-36 health survey can be summarized into two summary scores, the physical and mental component summary scores. Different versions and approaches to the scoring of the SF-36 are available; users should investigate the choices available and understand the advantages and disadvantages of each option. The 36 items are distributed by the Medical Outcomes Trust as the **SF-36 Health Survey** (versions 1.0 and 2.0 now distributed by qmetric), by RAND as the **RAND 36-Item Health Survey 1.0,** by the Health Outcomes Institute as the **Health Status Questionnaire** (plus three depression screening items), and by the Psychological Corporation as the **RAND-36 Health Status Inventory (HSI).**

VALUE AND USE

The SF-36 survey has been described as the most widely used patient-based measure of health-related quality of life in the world. It was originally designed to measure health status in health policy evaluation and general population surveys. The SF-36 is also used as an outcome measure in conjunction with disease-specific measures in clinical practice and research. The SF-36 compares favorably to other health profile instruments, with extensive evidence on the conceptual and measurement model, reliability, validity, respondent and administrative burden, alternative forms, and cultural and language adaptations. It takes approximately 7 to 10 minutes to self-administer. Alternative forms are available as 1- and 4-week recall periods, with self-report, interviewer-based, and computer-based versions. The SF-36 is useful in comparing general and specific subgroups, comparing the relative burden of diseases, differentiating the health benefits produced by various interventions and treatments, and screening individual patients.

ISSUES

Users should be informed about several developments that are relevant to application and interpretation of the SF-36. The philosophic and pragmatic merits and shortcomings of different methodological approaches (i.e., oblique versus orthogonal factor rotations) to generating physical and mental summary scores continue to be debated in the literature. A preference-based single index using the SF-36 that allows cost-utility analysis (*see terms:* Cost-Utility Analysis, Health Utilities Index) to be performed has been explored. Ongoing research into computer adaptive testing and measurement precision is likely to lead to further refinements in the way that health status measures such as the SF-36 are applied and interpreted.

BIBLIOGRAPHY

Brazier J, Usherwood T, Harper R, Thomas K. Deriving a preference-based single index from the UK SF-36 Health Survey. *J Clin Epidemiol.* 1998;51:1115–1128.

Coons SJ, Rao S, Keininger DL, Hays RD. A comparative review of generic quality-of-life instruments. *Pharmacoeconomics.* 2000;17:13–35.

McDowell I, Newell C. *Measuring Health: A Guide to Rating Scales and Questionnaires.* 2nd ed. New York: Oxford University Press; 1996.

Ware JE Jr., Sherbourne CD. The MOS 36-Item Short-Form Health Survey (SF-36): conceptual framework and item selection. *Med Care.* 1992;30:473–483.

# Sickness Impact Profile (SIP)

## BRIEF DEFINITION

The **Sickness Impact Profile (SIP)** is a generic health status instrument that measures the physical, psychosocial, and behavioral impact of disease.

## EXPLANATION

The SIP measures health status using a checklist of 136 items describing behavioral effects of illness (e.g., "I walk shorter distances or stop to rest often"). The subject is asked to place a check mark next to only those items that describe him or her on that day and that are related to his or her health. The SIP items are divided into 12 categories, encompassing both physical and psychosocial dimensions. The physical dimension consists of three categories: ambulation, mobility, and body care and movement. The psychosocial dimension consists of four categories: social interaction, alertness behavior, emotional behavior, and communication. There are also five independent categories: sleep and rest, eating, work, home management, and recreation and pastimes. The SIP score may be calculated as a profile with each of the 12 categories scored separately, as two dimension scores (e.g., physical and psychosocial) or as a single total (index) score. Scores range from 0 to 100, with higher scores reflecting a lower level of functioning.

## VALUE AND USE

The measurement properties of the SIP have been evaluated extensively, and it is widely regarded as a valid and reliable instrument. Like other generic questionnaires (e.g., the SF-36), the SIP was developed for use with different patient populations and, therefore is particularly useful for comparing the relative impact of different diseases and their treatment. The SIP is also a popular assessment tool because it produces a total score as well as individual scores for each of 12 categories of health status. The total score provides a means of summarizing the overall effect, while the individual category scores produce a more detailed picture, or profile, of the impact of a disease or treatment. To date, the SIP has been used to evaluate diverse patient populations including cardiovascular, gastrointestinal, neurologic, respiratory, and rheumatoid arthritis.

## ISSUES

When a health status measure is selected, the properties of the instrument that are most important depend on the primary purpose of the study. While generic instruments such as the SIP facilitate comparisons across a broad range of patient populations, they also tend to have less responsiveness—that is, are less sensitive to change—than a disease-specific instrument. For this reason, disease-specific questionnaires are often preferred for evaluating treatment effects—for example, in a clinical trial.

Another consideration in choosing a health status questionnaire is the practicality of administration. In this regard, the SIP has both advantages and disadvantages. Because it can be either self-administered or interviewer-administered, the SIP can be used in situations in which one or the other is required. Because the SIP is valid as an interviewer-administered questionnaire, it can be completed over the telephone or used with subjects whose physical disabilities make it difficult or impossible to complete a written questionnaire. The SIP can also be used in situations in which self-administration is the only viable option (e.g., in a mail survey study). The length of the SIP (136 items) may be prohibitive for some studies, requiring 20–30 minutes to complete when administered by an interviewer. Some work has been done to develop a shorter version of the questionnaire, but it has not yet received the same level of endorsement as the original version.

A third consideration is the availability of the SIP in languages other than English and cultures other than American. Although the copyright holders (MOS, Johns-Hopkins) do not currently recognize nonEnglish versions, they do offer tips for translating the SIP. A review of the medical literature shows that researchers have already tested translated versions (e.g., Spanish, Dutch).

BIBLIOGRAPHY

Bergner M, Bobbitt RA, Carter WB, Gilson BS. The Sickness Impact Profile: development and final revision of a health status measure. *Med Care.* 1981;19:787–805.

Bergner M, Bobbitt RA, Kressel S, et al. The Sickness Impact Profile: conceptual formulation and methodology for the development of a health status measure. *Int J Health Serv.* 1976;6:393–415.

De Bruin AF, De Witte LP. Sickness Impact Profile: the state of the art of a generic functional status measure. *Soc Sci Med.* 1992;358:1003–1014.

# Statistics in Pharmacoeconomics

**Descriptive Statistics**
**Inferential Statistics**
**Parametric Tests**
**Nonparametric Tests**

## BRIEF DEFINITION

**Statistics** can be described as the study of how to collect, organize, analyze, and interpret information, especially numerical information. In most real-life situations, important questions to be addressed involve incomplete information. The process of drawing good, reliable conclusions from incomplete information is central to the study of statistics.

## EXPLANATION

There are two primary divisions of the field of statistics: **descriptive statistics** and **inferential statistics**. The process of describing information using descriptive statistics, such as measures of central tendency (e.g., mean) and measures of dispersion (e.g., variance), is referred to as exploratory data analysis. This approach is also used to identify extreme scores, or oddly shaped distributions of scores. Although exploratory data analysis is an important process for understanding data in detail, we are often concerned with drawing inferences about a population.

There are two primary approaches to statistical inference: the Bayesian approach and the frequentist approach (*see term:* Bayesian Analysis). Bayesian approach is a branch of statistics based on Bayes' theorem. Bayesian inference does not use $P$-values and generally does not test hypotheses. It requires one to formally specify a probability distribution encapsulating the prior knowledge about, say, a treatment effect. The state of prior knowledge can be specified as "no knowledge" by using a flat distribution. Once the prior distribution is specified, the data are used to modify the prior state of knowledge to obtain the postexperiment state of knowledge. Final probabilities computed in the Bayesian framework are probability distributions for the treatment effects and can be used to estimate credible intervals for the treatment effect.

The most common approach to statistical inference, however, is the frequentist approach. The frequentist approach is also called the sampling approach, as it considers the distribution of statistics from hypothetical repeated samples from the same population. This approach uses hypothesis testing, type I and type II errors, significance level, power, confidence limits, $P$-values, and adjustment of $P$-values for testing multiple hypotheses from the same study. Final probabilities computed using frequentist methods (i.e., $P$-values) are probabilities of obtaining values of statistics.

## VALUE AND USE

In the frequentist approach, the statistical procedures involve both estimation of one or more parameters of the distribution of scores in the population(s) from which the data were sampled and assumptions concerning the shape of that distribution. For example, the t-test makes use of the sample variance ($s^2$) as an estimate of the population variance ($\sigma^2$) and also requires the assumption that the population from which the data were sampled is normal. Tests that make specific assumptions about the distribution of the data or specific assumptions about model parameters are referred to as **parametric tests**. Examples include the t-test and the Pearson product-moment linear correlation test.

There is a class of tests, however, that does not rely on parameter estimation and/or distribution assumptions. Such tests are usually referred to as **nonparametric tests** or distribution-free tests. Nonparametric tests for ordinal or continuous variables are typically based on the ranks of the data values. Such tests are unaffected by any one–one transformation of the data (e.g., by taking logs). If the data are not normal, a rank transformation can be more efficient than the corresponding parametric test. Examples of nonparametric tests include the two-sample Wilcoxon-Mann-Whitney test, the one-sample Wilcoxon signed rank test (usually used for paired data) and the Spearman, Kendall, or Somers rank correlation tests.

ISSUES

The major disadvantage attributed to nonparametric tests is their lower power relative to the corresponding parametric test. In general, when the assumptions of the parametric test are met, the distribution-free test requires more observations than does the comparable parametric test for the same level of power. Thus, for a given set of data, the parametric test is more likely to lead to rejection of a false null hypothesis than is the corresponding distribution-free test. Moreover, even when the distribution assumptions are violated to a moderate degree, the parametric tests are thought to maintain their advantage.

BIBLIOGRAPHY

Kendall M, Gibbons JD. *Rank Correlation Methods.* New York: Oxford University Press; 1990.

Spilker B, ed. *Quality of Life and Pharmacoeconomics in Clinical Trials.* New York: Raven Press; 1996.

Tukey JW. *Exploratory Data Analysis.* Reading, Mass: Addison-Wesley; 1977.

# Time-to-Event Models
Survival Analysis
Censoring
Survival Functions
Life Table
Log-Rank Test
Cox Regression Model
Proportional Hazards Modeling

BRIEF DEFINITION

**Time-to-event models** are models in which the main outcome is the time from the beginning of follow-up on a participant until an event of interest occurs. This model is often referred to as a **survival analysis**, because they were initially developed to analyze situations where the event of interest was patient death. However, the methodology can refer to any event occurring differentially over time in two or more groups.

EXPLANATION

Time-to-event models can analyze and compare the occurrence of an event over time. Data about whether and when the event of interest occurred is needed from each subject. Because some subjects may leave the study before the event occurs or the data collection period may end before all subjects have experienced the event, time-to-event analysis uses **censoring** to account for the incomplete information.

Typically, the probability of an event occurring changes over time. For example, if a patient has just undergone surgery, the likelihood of discharge from the hospital may be small; but as time goes on and healing occurs, the likelihood of discharge increases. The conditional probability of an event occurring at any point in time, given that it has not yet occurred, is estimated from the study data. These estimates are called **survival functions**.

Analysis involves two main steps: estimating the distribution of the survival data to calculate a survival function followed by comparison of survival curves for two or more alternatives to determine whether they have different survival functions.

There are two methods for estimating the distribution of the survival data over time and calculating the survival function. The **life table** or actuarial method summarizes how many subjects have had the event and how many have not at each time point. It provides an estimate of median time-to-event (when 50% of subjects have experienced the event). The product-limit method produces Kaplan-Meier curves, which are really step functions, which plot the likelihood of survival against time. Survival refers to absence of the event, whether the event is death or another change in condition. Every time an event or censoring of a subject occurs, the step function drops.

Once survival functions are calculated, the differences between groups may be assessed using a **log-rank test**, which compares the likelihood of survival in each group across the whole span of time. Other tests are available which put more weight on some parts of the curve than others.

To assess the impact of other variables on survival time, a **Cox regression model** is used. For each additional variable of interest, such as age or gender, the model provides an estimate of the relative risk for members of the cohort adjusted for other factors in the model. A more sophisticated model can include time-varying independent variables (e.g., lab measures taken repeatedly over the course of the study). This analytic approach assumes proportional hazards across treatment groups and is sometimes referred to as **proportional hazards modeling**.

## Value and Use

Time-to-event models have many applications in health outcomes research and pharmacoeconomics, such as assessing differences in groups on time to discharge from hospital, time to a change in prescription, time to development of a new condition (e.g., adverse event or recovery), or time to recurrence of the disease being studied. They may be used to analyze differences in treatment effects on disease progression in chronic diseases such as AIDS.

## Issues

Censoring of an observation is an inherent issue in time-to-event modeling. An observation is censored when it can no longer be determined whether the subject experienced the event or not. For example, if a patient has not had the event and data collection is discontinued, the observation is censored at the end of the study. Some observations will be censored prior to the end of the study due to other events that preclude the event of interest (e.g., the event of interest is discharge from hospital but patient dies). The statistical methods for analyzing this data assume that censoring is noninformative. Noninformative censoring implies that the reason for censoring the data was not due to something that could influence the likelihood of the event occurring. In the above example, patient death is informative censoring because the patient never had a chance of reaching discharge. Informative censoring is a difficult matter to detect and handle. In cases such as this, it is prudent to define the event in advance to include possible causes of informative censoring. For example, the event could be defined as time to death *or* discharge from hospital. The analysis can then be run once with events combined and once with them separated to determine whether results are robust to the definition used.

## Bibliography

Allison, PD. *Survival Analysis Using the SAS System.* Cary, Ill: SAS Institute; 1995.

Kleinbaum DG. *Survival Analysis: A Self-Learning Text.* New York: Springer Statistics in the Health Sciences; 1996.

# Uncertainty

## BRIEF DEFINITION

**Uncertainty** occurs when the true value of a parameter (x) is unknown, reflecting the fact that knowledge or measurement is not perfect. Expressing the uncertainty surrounding the true value of a parameter (x) involves identifying the range of values that could be reasonably attributed to x.

## EXPLANATION

Uncertainty is distinct from variability, which reflects known differences in parameter values associated with identifiable differences in circumstances (e.g., different practice patterns in different geographical areas, or differing treatment effects based on age and/or sex). However, the distinction between uncertainty and variability often depends upon the question that is being addressed. For example, in a model of antibiotic treatment, resistance rates could be represented as uncertain within a geographical community and variable between communities. That is, there is knowledge that identifiably different communities have different resistance rates, although the actual value of the resistance in any community is itself not known precisely.

In pharmacoeconomics, there are various sources of uncertainty including methodological, structural, parameter, and stochastic uncertainty.

Methodological uncertainty reflects uncertainty regarding the analytic methods used within an economic evaluation. This source of uncertainty may include, for example, uncertainty relating to the discount rate employed, the method used for the valuation of resources, or the method used for the valuation of health outcomes.

Structural uncertainty reflects uncertainty concerning the structure and assumptions employed within an analysis—for example, the method used to incorporate the relative risk of treatment or the method used to extrapolate results beyond the period of measurement. This type of uncertainty is particularly prevalent within analyses based upon models.

Parameter uncertainty reflects the uncertainty surrounding parameters within a model—for example, uncertainty surrounding the effectiveness of a technology, the utility associated with a health state, or the resource use associated with a technology.

Stochastic or first order uncertainty reflects uncertainty within a population (e.g., the different cost associated with patients within a clinical trial, the different number and type of events experienced by patients within a population).

## VALUE AND USE

In order for economic evaluations to be useful for decision-making purposes, the results should include some estimate of the impact of uncertainty upon the payoffs (costs, effects, cost-effectiveness) attributable to a technology and ultimately the uncertainty surrounding the decision.

Sensitivity analysis is the method used to investigate the impact of uncertainty upon payoffs and decisions (*see term:* Sensitivity Analysis). Commonly used techniques include one-way sensitivity analysis and multi-way sensitivity analysis; threshold and scenario analysis; analysis of extremes and probabilistic sensitivity analysis. Regardless of the nature of the sensitivity analysis, the practice involves substitution of values and observation of the impact upon the payoffs. Within the process the substitution can affect parameter values, assumptions, or methods (e.g., a reanalysis using a different discount rate over a shorter follow-up period or employing a different set of price weights).

Methodological and structural uncertainty is handled through deterministic sensitivity analysis. One-way and multi-way sensitivity analysis involves substituting different values for one or more of the parameters, assumptions, or methods used within the analysis. Analysis of extremes involves changing all parameters to extreme values (either best or worst case) simultaneously. Threshold analysis involves identifying the level of one or more parameters, assumptions, or methods at which the decision switches.

Variability is handled through scenario analysis. The process, a form of multi-way analysis, involves simultaneously substituting the parameter values and assumptions associated with an identifiable subgroup of interest.

Parameter uncertainty is handled through either deterministic or probabilistic sensitivity analysis. A probabilistic sensitivity analysis involves a second order Monte Carlo simulation, and the results reflect uncertainty at the population level. The process involves specifying a probability distribution for each of the parameters of interest to fully reflect the parameter uncertainty. Each distribution represents both the range of values that the parameter can take as well as the probability that it takes any particular value. At each iteration within the simulation, a value is selected for each parameter from its individual probability distribution, the analysis is repeated, and the result is identified. Each iteration represents a realization of the uncertainty that exists in the analysis as characterized by the probability distributions. Within a Monte Carlo simulation, this process is repeated a large number of times to propagate the uncertainty and results in a distribution of possible payoffs associated with the technologies of interest. This type of analysis is a second order simulation and provides an estimate of the second order uncertainty (i.e., the uncertainty in the mean or population level values). This is distinct from a first order Monte Carlo simulation, which provides an estimate of the within-population uncertainty. A first order simulation involves simulating the experience of each patient individually, generating a pathway for each patient with associated payoffs.

Within a trial analysis, first order uncertainty is expressed using measures of dispersion (e.g., the standard deviation, variance, inter-quartile range). An estimate of the second order uncertainty can be obtained through bootstrapping the sample data.

While an assessment of within-population (first order) uncertainty may be of interest, it is the level of second order uncertainty that is important to the policymaker, who is concerned with examining the implications of policy at a macro (population) level.

In order to express the uncertainty associated with a decision, it is necessary to incorporate a decision rule into the analysis. In pharmacoeconomics, the standard decision rule employed involves comparing the incremental cost-effectiveness ratio (*see term:* Cost-Effective Analysis) (ICER) with a predefined threshold value ($\lambda$). A technology is then adopted if it is associated with an ICER that is less than the threshold. Decision uncertainty is the uncertainty surrounding a decision made upon this basis and can be presented for various levels of the threshold using cost-effectiveness acceptability curves. It must be noted that decision uncertainty can be very different from uncertainty surrounding payoffs, due to the addition of a decision rule (in this case $\lambda$). For example, a technology may be associated with very large uncertainty surrounding the costs and effects that are attributable to it without any associated decision uncertainty. This would be the case where the entire range of costs as negative and the entire range of effects as positive, as the technology would dominate over the entire range.

## ISSUES

Deterministic sensitivity analysis can provide an initial, qualitative assessment of uncertainty and currently prevails in the literature. However, the nature of deterministic sensitivity analyses means that they ignore (one-way) or exaggerate (analysis of extremes) the interaction between parameters, providing results that are qualitative and difficult to interpret. Indeed, it is only when a sensitivity analysis is shown to have no impact upon the decision that the results are usable. A complete assessment of uncertainty requires a probabilistic sensitivity analysis. This type of analysis appropriately handles interactions between parameters and provides interpretable, quantitative results. In addition, in the presence of nonlinearities within model structures (for example discounting), only a probabilistic analysis provides a good estimate of the expected payoffs associated with health technologies.

However, probabilistic analysis can only be used to represent uncertainty in parameters; it cannot and should not be used to represent uncertainty surrounding assumptions, methods, or structure. The methods of deterministic sensitivity analysis remain the main method for handling uncertainty in these areas.

## BIBLIOGRAPHY

Briggs AH. Handling uncertainty in economic evaluation and presenting the results. In: Drummond M, McGuire A, eds. *Economic Evaluation in Health Care: Merging Theory with Practice.* Oxford, UK: Oxford University Press; 2001.

Briggs AH, Sculpher M, Buxton M. Uncertainty in the economic evaluation of health care technologies: the role of sensitivity analysis. *Health Economics.* 1994;3:95–104.

Hunink M, Glasziou P, Siegel J, Weeks J, Pliskin J, Elstein A, Weinstein M. Variability and uncertainty. In: Hunink M, Glasziou P, Siegel J, Weeks J, Pliskin J, Elstein A, Weinstein M, eds. *Decision Making in Health and Medicine. Integrating Evidence and Values.* Cambridge, UK: Cambridge University Press; 2002.

# Utility

## BRIEF DEFINITION

A **utility** is a quantitative expression of an individual's preference for, or desirability of, a particular state of health under conditions of uncertainty.

## EXPLANATION

Utilities are numbers that represent the strength of an individual's preference for different health outcomes under conditions of uncertainty. The conventional utility scale has a utility of 0.0 for dead and a utility of 1.0 for complete health. States worse than dead can have negative utilities.

Utility scores can be assigned by direct measurement using techniques like the standard gamble and the time trade-off (*see term:* Utility Measurement). Alternatively, the scores can be assigned indirectly by using a utility-weighted index (*see terms:* EuroQol, Health Utilities Index, Quality of Well-Being Scale).

When scores are assigned by the standard gamble, which involves uncertainty, they are true utilities. When scores are assigned by other methods that do not involve uncertainty (e.g., time trade-off, visual analog scale) they are technically not utilities, but values. Utilities and values are both preferences. Readers should be aware, however, that many writers fail to make these distinctions and often use the term "utility" to cover both types of preferences—utilities and values.

Utility scores reflect preferences for the whole health state and thus integrate the effects of efficacy (improved health) and side effects (adverse events). Utility scores are used as the quality weights when computing a quality-adjusted life year (QALY) (*see term:* Quality-Adjusted Life Year [QALY]). This allows morbidity and mortality changes to be combined into one single weighted measure, the QALY.

Utility scores from direct measurement can be provided by patients, clinicians or the general population. Utility scores built into the scoring formulae of utility-weighted indexes are all provided by the general population.

In clinical trials, utility measures can be valuable because patients combine positive and negative effects of an intervention into one single value on the utility scale. The two approaches in a clinical trial are to measure utilities directly using a utility measurement instrument (i.e., to ask subjects to assign a value to their overall health using a standard gamble technique or a time trade-off method) or indirectly using a utility-weighted index (i.e., to classify patients into categories based on their responses to questions about their functional status and to score the result with the utility scoring formula provided with the instrument). The methods are not mutually exclusive and both can be used in the same study.

## VALUE AND USE

Utility measurements offer a patient the possibility to value different aspects of treatment and outcomes. Hard scientific end points such as survival and laboratory measurements can be supplemented with subjective results such as quality of life and incorporated in the final choice of the patient between different therapies. Utility measurements can also be used in cost-utility analysis (*see term:* Cost-Utility Analysis), a tool in the decision-making process for the allocation of financial resources to health care interventions.

## ISSUES

Controversy exists regarding the question "whose preferences should be used?"—that is, the preferences of the patients who have actually experienced a particular health state or those of a representative community sample who have not. Evidence suggests that people experiencing a condition may attach a higher value to it. The US Public Health Service Panel on Cost-Effectiveness in Health and Medicine has suggested that public policy decisions involving the allocation of limited resources should incorporate the utilities of the general public obtained through use of preference-classification systems rather than those of the affected patients. On the other hand, clinical decisions for particular patients should be made using their utilities.

## BIBLIOGRAPHY

Bakker CH, Rutten-van Molken M, van Doorslaer E, et al. Health related utility measurement in rheumatology: an introduction. *Patient Educ Couns.* 1993;20:145–152.

Gabriel SE, Kneeland TS, Melton LJ, et al. Health-related quality of life in economic evaluations for osteoporosis: whose values should we use? *Med Decis Making.* 1999;19:141–148.

Gold MR, Siegel JE, Russell LB, Weinstein ME. *Cost-Effectiveness in Health Medicine.* New York: Oxford University Press; 1996.

Revicki DA, Kaplan RM. Relationship between psychometric and utility-based approaches to the measurement of health-related quality of life. *Qual Life Res.* 1993;2:477–487.

# Utility Measurement

**Standard Gamble (SG)**
**Time Trade-Off (TTO)**
**Visual Analog Scale (VAS)**

## BRIEF DEFINITION

**Utility measurement** is a method of querying an individual in order to measure the strength of preference that the individual has for an outcome (e.g., a health state), and to represent that preference by a quantitative score called a utility (*see term:* Utility). The more preferred the outcome, the higher the utility score. Two widely used methods for measuring such preferences are the **standard gamble** (SG) and the **time trade-off** (TTO). In both methods the individual expresses her or his lack of preference for the outcome by indicating the maximum loss that he or she would accept to avoid the outcome. In the standard gamble, the loss is expressed as a risk of a specified bad outcome, often death. In the time trade-off, the loss is expressed as a reduction in healthy life expectancy.

## EXPLANATION

Individuals have preferences for alternative health outcomes (e.g., prefer health state A to health state B) and can express them. The health outcomes for which preferences are measured can be simple outcomes (e.g., single health states), complex outcomes (e.g., a profile of health states over a lifetime), or even health programs. The preferences can be measured on an ordinal scale or a cardinal scale. An ordinal scale is simply a rank ordering of the outcomes. A cardinal scale is a continuous numeric scale. The particular type of cardinal scale used for the measurement of preferences in health is an interval scale. An interval scale is like a temperature scale (Fahrenheit, Celsius) in that any two states can be given arbitrary scores (freezing, boiling) and all other states are then measured relative to these two. In the most common version of health utilities, death is given a score of 0.0, perfect health is given a score of 1.0, and all other outcomes are scored relative to these two. Note that this does not preclude outcomes or states worse than death with scores less than zero.

The standard gamble (SG) and the time trade-off (TTO) are two widely used methods to measure an individual's preferences for health outcomes on an interval scale. The SG is based directly on expected utility theory as first postulated by von Neumann and Morgenstern, and is particularly designed for use in problems in which the outcomes are uncertain (e.g., health problems). In all fields but health (e.g., business, military, environment) the SG is the overwhelmingly preferred method to measure utilities. In early applications in health, the SG was cumbersome to administer and the TTO was developed as an alternative. Unlike the SG, the TTO does not measure preferences under uncertainty (there are no probabilities in the TTO question), and as such, the preference scores from the TTO are technically values, not utilities. Methods for the SG have now improved to the point where it is no longer difficult to administer, and both techniques are widely used. Many researchers consider the SG better because of its direct applicability to a world of uncertainty, while others disagree.

In the SG, an individual expresses his or her preference by choosing between two alternatives. For example, an individual who prefers A to B to C would be asked to choose between one alternative in which outcome B would be received with certainty and a second alternative in which outcome A would be received with probability $p$ and outcome C with probability $(1 - p)$. The probability $p$ would then be varied until the individual was indifferent between these two choices. The indifference probability is used to calculate the utility that the individual has for outcome B relative to the utilities for outcomes A and C. Details of the method are widely available.

In the TTO, an individual expresses his or her preference also by choosing between two alternatives. For example, an individual who preferred perfect health to B would be asked to choose between one alternative in which outcome B would be received with certainty for the remaining life expectancy $t$ and a second alternative in which perfect health would be received but for a shortened life expectancy of length $x < t$. The duration $x$ would then be varied until the individual was indifferent between these two choices. The ratio $x/t$ is the TTO value score for outcome B on a scale where immediate death is 0.0 and perfect health for the lifetime duration $t$ is 1.0. Details of the TTO method are available in the same references listed above for SG.

### Value and Use

Despite the distinction described above between utilities and values, it is common in the health field to use the term "utilities" as an umbrella word to cover both. We do so from here on in this section.

Utilities may be measured directly or indirectly. Direct measurement requires the use of SG or TTO (or sometimes other alternatives such as a **visual analog scale [VAS]**, or person trade-offs). These techniques are often interviewer-administered, and thus costly and time-consuming, although self-administered versions and computer-interactive versions are increasingly becoming available.

Indirect measurement, on the other hand, is much easier. It involves a simple, often self-administered, questionnaire that determines the respondent's health status. The utility is calculated from a scoring formula that is part of the instrument. The scoring formula, in turn, is based on community preferences as measured by the SG, the TTO, or the VAS. The three most widely used instruments are the Health Utilities Index (*see term*: Health Utilities Index), which is based on SG measurements, the EuroQol EQ-5D (*see term*: EuroQol), which is based on TTO measurements, and the Quality of Well-Being Scale (*see term*: Quality of Well-Being Scale), which is based on VAS measurements.

Because utility measurement is relatively new, many existing data sets do not contain utility data. However, they sometimes contain other data that can be mapped into utilities as a second best approach. Mapping routines have been proposed or are under development for the US Annual Health Interview Survey, the US National Health and Nutritional Examination Survey and the Short Form 36.

When utility scores are measured on the conventional health utility scale where dead = 0.0 and perfect health = 1.0, the scores are appropriate for calculating quality-adjusted life years and for use in cost-utility analysis.

### Issues

There is considerable debate about whose preferences should count—those of the informed general public (community preferences) or those of patients. For program evaluation and funding decisions, the recommendation is that community preferences are the most relevant, although it is generally conceded that patients' preferences, if different, should also be investigated and discussed. For clinical decision making for an individual patient, the patient's preferences of that particular patient are the most relevant.

Different ways of measuring utility give different results. This is true both for direct measurement (e.g., SG verus TTO) and for indirect measurements (e.g., HUI versus EQ-5D). This is a major concern because it makes it difficult to compare across studies that use different methods. On the other hand, different populations (different respondents) tend not to make much difference. This is encouraging, because it suggests that utilities measured on one group (e.g., residents of a particular city or province) can be applied to other groups (e.g., those elsewhere in the same country, or even those in other countries).

## BIBLIOGRAPHY

Drummond MF, O'Brien BJ, Stoddart GL, Torrance GW. *Methods for the Economic Evaluation of Health Care Programmes.* 2nd ed. Oxford, UK: Oxford University Press; 1997.

Furlong W, Feeny DH, Torrance GW, Barr R, Horsman J. Guide to Design and Development of Health-State Utility Instrumentation. Centre for Health Economics and Policy Analysis, Working Paper No. 90-9. Hamilton, Canada: McMaster University; 1990.

Torrance GW. Measurement of health-state utilities for economic appraisal: A review. *J Health Econ.* 1986;5:1–30.

# Validity
Face Validity
Content Validity
Criterion Validity
Construct Validity
Structural Validity
Process Validity
Outcome Validity
Validation

## BRIEF DEFINITION
**Validity** describes how well a measurement tool or economic evaluation allows us to infer something about the true nature and value of the object or system being considered.

## EXPLANATION
As defined here, validity may refer to the measurement of data or economic evaluations. Measurement is used to place a value on variables; economic evaluation models are used to represent how costs and consequences of alternatives are used in actual medical practice. Both are important in pharmacoeconomics and outcomes research.

## Validity in Measuring Data

Strictly speaking, validity is not a characteristic of a measurement tool; it is a characteristic of the inferences that are made about the scores that the tool produced. However, validity is commonly described as how well a tool measures what it says it is going measure. Either way, one needs to consider the validity of the data produced within the context of the population and setting in which it is produced.

When an instrument appears to measure what it says it will measure to the person being measured, it is said to have **face validity**. Face validity is used in survey research to describe how potential respondents view the questionnaire. Many researchers consider this aspect of validity to be too vague and subjective and have abandoned the concept. In contrast, expert opinion is used to determine whether an instrument has **content validity** (i.e., the items in the questionnaire should measure what they are designed to measure). **Criterion validity** may be tested when the results obtained by one instrument can be verified through an independent observation or another instrument that has already been validated. **Construct validity** is the degree to which the instrument measures the underlying trait of interest. The underlying trait is usually latent (i.e., not observable). In outcomes research, such traits include satisfaction and health status.

## Validity in Economic Evaluations

Models are used in economic evaluations to represent real systems. The extent to which a model does so may be described by several other validity terms. The degree to which an evaluation contains the type of resource (input) variables that represent usual medical practice for a given type of clinical setting is called **structural validity**. The degree to which the evaluation models a series of clinical interventions to show when and how the resources are used in a manner that mirrors actual practice is **process validity**. In contrast, **outcome validity** is the degree to which the estimated costs and consequences of the model agree with the observed costs and consequences of actual practice. This may also be described as predictive validity.

### Value and Use

Validity is an important characteristic of measurements and models used in pharmacoeconomics and outcomes research. If the data used for decision making are not measured appropriately or are not analyzed in models that represent real systems, the risk of reaching inappropriate conclusions exists. The popular adage "garbage in, garbage out" applies here.

Valid measurement is most difficult to determine when the variables are not explicit. Latent traits such as knowledge, satisfaction, and health status are important outcome measures that cannot be directly measured. Validity is most frequently evaluated and discussed in the outcomes research literature where the results of the development and adaptation of health status and satisfaction questionnaires are presented.

The process of testing and assuring validity in an instrument is termed **validation**. There are a number of methods that can be used to evaluate the validity of an instrument (see Bibliography listings for more information). In general, content validity is always considered important since it involves the clinical sensibility of the instrument. When developing an instrument to measure a particular aspect of HRQOL there may be little prior knowledge about the constructs and dimensionality; in this case, assuring construct validity is very important.

### Issues

Validity is not reliability. Reliability is the ability of a measurement tool to produce consistent scores when the same trait is measured several times. It is possible to get consistent, reliable scores from an instrument that is not valid. However, to be valid, a measurement tool should be able to produce reliably consistent scores (i.e., it should be reliable).

The traditional concept of validity in psychometric research has been criticized and modified by several researchers (Pedhazur and Schmelkin 1991; Messick 1995).

Because validity is not a property of the instrument itself, it is important to perform a new validation process each time an instrument is used in a new setting or population. While the instrument does not change, the meaning of the scores in the new population may. Reports of efforts to adapt and translate health status surveys into different languages and cultures provide an excellent example of this principle.

Instruments are usually validated by a series of studies, not a single study. When evaluating an instrument, researchers should look at the body of literature describing the populations and situations in which it was used and the methods by which it was administered (e.g., written questionnaire, telephone interview).

The bottom line is "good pharmacoeconomics research requires both valid models and valid measurements." If either the data measurement or the model is not valid, the researcher risks reaching a false conclusion.

## BIBLIOGRAPHY

Fayers PM, Machin D. *Quality of Life: Assessment, Analysis, and Interpretation.* West Sussex, UK: John Wiley & Sons Ltd; 2000.

Messick S. Validity. In: Linn RL, ed. *Educational Measurement, Third Edition. National Council on Measurement in Education and American Council on Education, Series in Higher Education.* Phoenix, Ariz: ORYX; 1993.

Messick S. Validity of psychological assessment: Validation of inferences from person's responses and performance as scientific inquiry into scoring meaning. *Am Psychol.* 1995;9:741–749.

Pedhazur EJ, Schmelkin LP. *Measurement, Design and Analysis: An Integrated Approach.* Hillsdale, Mich: Erlbaum Associates Publishers; 1991.

Streiner DL, Norman GR. *Health Measurement Scales: A Practical Guide to their Development and Use.* 2nd ed. New York: Oxford University Press; 1995.

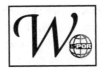

# Welfare Economics

Potential Pareto Improvement
Maximin Approach
Welfarist Approach
Extra-Welfarist Approach

## BRIEF DEFINITION

**Welfare economics** is the study of the well-being of members of a society as a group and involves both normative and positive analysis. Economic analysis cannot determine the objectives of society, but once those objectives are determined, it can shed light on the appropriateness of different policies as means of achieving them. The types of policy which might be assessed in this way include government taxation and expenditure, tariffs, and industrial organization. Welfare economics provides the conceptual basis for economic evaluation techniques such as cost-benefit analysis, which are used in the health sector (*see term:* Cost-Benefit Analysis).

## EXPLANATION

The economic consequences of policies are customarily assessed in terms of efficiency and equity. Welfare economics has a normative basis since value judgments are needed on how these terms should be measured and their relative importance to society before any assessment of policy options can take place. Two common value judgments in welfare economics are that social ranking of policies should be based on the rankings of individuals, and that an individual is the best judge of his or her own welfare. The subjective nature of this judgment of personal welfare means that an individual can indicate preferences between different situations, but it makes aggregate societal comparison of welfare difficult. The only situation in which a change can be declared indisputably beneficial is when at least one individual feels better off and all other people feel no worse off (known to economists as the Pareto criterion). These conditions are very restrictive and few policy changes can meet this criterion. A modified form, was developed to widen its practical application. In the modified form, a compensation test is applied to determine whether those gaining from a policy change could compensate the losers to the extent that they no longer feel worse off. If the gainers can do this and still feel better off after doing so, the change is considered a **potential Pareto improvement**. The compensation does not have to take place for the criterion to be met, which immediately raises the issue of distribution of economic benefits.

Neoclassical microeconomics demonstrates that under certain assumptions, individual choice and competitive markets will produce a level and distribution of welfare that cannot be improved using the Pareto principle. However, there are many such allocations, each with different distributional implications, and the Pareto criterion offers no means of choosing among them. To include considerations of income distribution requires the adoption of a social welfare function based on some ethical principle. Examples include the egalitarian **maximin approach**, which ranks options on the basis of how much they give to the least well-off in society. Use of willingness-to-pay (*see term:* Contingent Valuation) by beneficiaries as a method of judging the social value of a policy assumes acceptance of the current distribution of income.

## ISSUES

In health and health care policy, issues of equity have traditionally been seen as important, and policymakers in all countries have been reluctant to leave health care provision to the marketplace. The main reasons for this are a belief that the asymmetry of information between consumers and providers prevents the achievement of efficient output (often referred to as market failure), and that ability-to-pay should not determine access to necessary health care.

The techniques of economic evaluation have been developed to help decision makers compare the economic benefits of different policies in situations in which the data observed from competitive markets do not provide a complete measure of the social benefits and costs of policies (e.g., the benefits to the whole population from immunization programs targeted at specific groups). However, there are difficulties with the use of these techniques in the health field because the main benefits of health policies—reduced mortality and morbidity—are not easily expressed in monetary terms. The economic methods most closely based on economic theory (e.g., cost-benefit analysis) may not be accepted by other professional groups involved in health policymaking.

Economists now distinguish between **welfarist approach** and **extra-welfarist approach** to evaluation in health care. The welfarist approach follows conventional economic theory and takes account of the impact of policy on the total welfare of individuals, not just that related directly to their health status. This would take account of the costs (in time and inconvenience as well as money) borne by patients in obtaining treatment as well as their financial benefits from restoration of health. This requires the use of cost-benefit analysis with nonfinancial benefits, such as the value of health per se, evaluated using contingent valuation techniques such as willingness-to-pay (*see term:* Contingent Valuation).

The extra-welfarist approach treats health-gain as the objective of health policy and ignores nonhealth-related factors. This allows the use of cost-effectiveness analysis and cost-utility analysis to rank health projects with gains measured in terms of life-year, quality-adjusted life year, or healthy-year equivalent, with only the costs to the health system considered (*see terms:* Healthy-Year Equivalent, Quality-Adjusted Life Year [QALY]). Conventionally, the assumption is made that a unit of health gain accruing to any individual is worth the same to society. However, it is possible to introduce other value judgments by weighting benefits to certain groups. (This is also possible in the welfarist approach if willingness-to-pay is adjusted for ability-to-pay.) The two approaches may not produce the same result, as the policy that maximizes health gain—measured, for example, by quality-adjusted life years—may not be the one that produces the maximum welfare as perceived by the individuals affected.

Economic evaluation techniques are now routinely applied in health care decisions, often without regard to their origins and limitations. Welfare economics reminds us that all methods are based on value judgments and that the use of a method implies acceptance of the values on which it is based.

BIBLIOGRAPHY

Boadway RW, Bruce N. *Welfare Economics*. Oxford, UK: Basil Blackwell; 1984.

Hurley J. An overview of the normative economics of the health sector. In: Culyer AJ, Newhouse JP, eds. *Handbook of Health Economics*, volume 1A. Amsterdam: Elsevier; 2000.

# About the Editors

**Marc L. Berger,** MD, Vice President, US Human Health Outcomes Research and Management, Merck & Company, Inc.

Dr Berger obtained his MD degree from Johns Hopkins University School of Medicine. He completed an internal medicine residency at NYU-Bellevue Hospital in New York and a Liver Research Fellowship at the University of Texas Health Science Center at Dallas-Southwestern Medical School. Prior to joining Merck, he was on the faculty of the University of Cincinnati School of Medicine. While at Merck, Dr Berger has held various positions of responsibility for Phase II to Phase IV clinical trials, outcomes research studies, and disease management programs. He is currently vice president of outcomes research and management (ORM) in the US Human Health Division, Merck's Company, Inc., West Point, PA, USA. ORM is an interdisciplinary department of physicians, economists, epidemiologists, pharmacists, psychologists, and other professionals that (1) conducts health services/outcomes research studies examining the gap between current patterns of health care delivery and what would be considered optimal according to evidence-based medicine; (2) is responsible for the research and development of disease management tools and programs offered as value-added services to large health care providers; and (3) conducts research and analyses that demonstrate the value of Merck products and of pharmaceutical innovation to payers, providers, and patients.

Dr Berger has coauthored numerous articles in outcomes research and health economics. His current research interests include health-related productivity, cost-effectiveness analysis, disease management, and the value of pharmaceutical innovation. He serves as a member of the editorial advisory boards of *Value in Health* and *Managed Healthcare* and as a member of the advisory board of the Program on the Economic Evaluation of Medical Technology (PEEMT) at the Harvard Center for Risk Analysis. Dr Berger is a trustee of the Occupational and Environmental Health Foundation and serves as chair of the Quality Initiatives Group of the National Pharmaceutical Council. He holds appointments as an adjunct senior fellow at the Leonard David Institute of Health Economics at the University of Pennsylvania and adjunct professor in the Department of Health Policy and Administration at the University of North Carolina at Chapel Hill School of Public Health.

**Kerstin (Chris) Bingefors,** PhD, Associate Professor, Uppsala University

Chris Bingefors is currently associate professor of pharmacoepidemiology at the Department of Pharmacy, Uppsala University, Uppsala, Sweden. She is also research director for the pharmacoepidemiology and pharmacoeconomics group at the same department. She received her MSc (Pharm) from the Faculty of Pharmacy in Uppsala and her PhD in Psychiatric Health Services Research from the Faculty of Medicine at Uppsala University. She is a research associate at the Department of Neuroscience, Psychiatry at the same university. She has also spent a year as associate professor at the University of Tromsö in northern Norway.

Dr Bingefors has authored and coauthored about 40 scientific articles and book chapters on epidemiology, health economics, quality of life, and compliance. After taking graduate courses in the United States, she was responsible for introducing and implementing public health, pharmacoepidemiology, and health economics in the Swedish pharmacy curriculum in the early eighties. Dr Bingefors received the Pharmaceutical Society award for excellence in teaching for her work. Dr Bingefors is very active in continuing professional education of physicians, dentists, nurses, and other health care staff. She has been active in many professional societies; among them are the Swedish Pharmaceutical Society, the Swedish Pharmaceutical Association (she is currently on the board), and the International Society for Pharmacoepidemiology, where she served on the board of directors from 1997 to 2000. She is currently serving as a director of the board of ISPOR. Her ISPOR activities also include work on the Awards Committee at several meetings, the core group for the ISPOR Research Excellence Award Task Force, and the core group for the Avedis Donabedian Lifetime Achievement Award and the European Meeting Abstract Review Committee.

Dr Bingefors' current interests include psychiatry, neurology, and dermatology, where she does research in epidemiology, HRQL, clinical and economic outcomes, compliance, and the population health impact of drug treatment. She is also developing gender-focused research within these areas.

### Edwin C. Hedblom, PharmD, Global Health Economics Manager, 3M

Edwin Hedblom is Global Health Economics Manager at 3M Medical in St. Paul, Minnesota, USA, and is responsible for health economic and reimbursement strategies for 3M Medical products worldwide.

Dr Hedblom's interests have been largely in the development, communication, and use of health economics and outcomes information by consumers, purchasers, and managers of health care.

He brings a unique perspective to the use of health economic information in the management and delivery of health care and the reimbursement decision-making process, as he has held positions in the managed care, consumer health, and pharmaceutical industries. In addition to his experience at 3M, Dr Hedblom has served as chief pharmacy officer for AARP Pharmacy Services and the chief pharmacy officer for Aetna US Healthcare. He has also served AstraZeneca as its global director for health economics and has held positions in the AstraZeneca integration, as well as having had roles in disease and patient management.

Dr Hedblom received his doctor of pharmacy and bachelor of pharmacy degrees from the University of Minnesota College of Pharmacy.

**Chris L. Pashos,** PhD, Vice President and Executive Director of HERQuLES, Abt Associates

Dr Pashos leads the HERQuLES Team at Abt Associates Inc., Cambridge, MA, USA. Abt Associates is a worldwide research and technical assistance organization with over 1000 staff, known for its portfolio of work as diverse as research and technical assistance to improve health care systems, the US national immunization survey, and clinical trial operations for an artificial implantable heart. The HERQuLES team provides a variety of research and strategic services to pharmaceutical, biotechnology, and medical device companies. Retrospective services include development of interactive economic models and analyses of US and European claims and other databases. Prospective studies include trials, observational studies, and patient and physician surveys to obtain data on the use of health care services and on the clinical, economic, and patient reported outcomes of that care. He has directed patient registries involving hundreds of thousands of patients across a variety of clinical indications and chaired a Biotechnology Industry Organization (BIO) panel on preapproval and postmarketing patient registries.

Dr Pashos joined Abt Associates in 1995, coming from the faculty of the Harvard Medical School Department of Health Care Policy. There, he directed the Harvard heart attack Patient Outcomes Research Team (PORT), one of the first four PORTs funded by the United States government to study the quality of health care. He also created and directed the Harvard Medical School Bridges Program, which brought together national policymakers, academic experts, and private decision makers to discuss critical health care issues. He has also consulted to governments in North America, Europe, Asia, and Africa and to international organizations, including the United Nations.

Having published in leading medical journals and lectured on the cost and value of health care, Dr Pashos has chaired the ISPOR Communications Committee, served as the associate editor for health policy of the *Journal of Clinical Outcomes Management*, and served on the editorial advisory board of *Value in Health*. He served as editor of the ISPOR Lexicon and is a recipient of the ISPOR Distinguished Service Award.

Dr Pashos earned his BS degree with distinction from the US Naval Academy and his MPP and PhD degrees in public policy from Harvard University.

**George W. Torrance,** PhD, Professor Emeritus, McMaster University

Dr Torrance received BASc and MBA degrees from the University of Toronto and a PhD in engineering from the State University of New York at Buffalo. He is professor emeritus of clinical epidemiology and biostatistics and of management science at McMaster University, Hamilton, Canada. He is affiliated with the Centre for Health Economics and Policy Analysis at McMaster University and the Centre for Evaluation of Medicines at St. Joseph's Hospital, Burlington, Ontario, Canada. In addition, he is vice president of Innovus Research Inc., a contract research organization with offices in Toronto, Boston, and London. Innovus undertakes outcomes research, economic evaluations, and clinical trials for the health care industry worldwide.

Dr Torrance's many publications include contributions to both the methods and applications of health economics. Methodological contributions include the use of utility theory and multi-attribute utility theory to measure preferences for health outcomes. Applications include neonatal intensive care, end-stage kidney disease, childhood cancer, post–myocardial infarction rehabilitation, prenatal diagnosis, arthritis, total knee replacement, workers' compensation board awards, the measurement of population health, and new drugs and devices for a wide variety of diseases. In addition, Dr Torrance and his colleagues developed the widely applied Health Utilities Index and operate Health Utilities Inc., a service center for users.

Dr Torrance has served as a local district health council member, a hospital board member, and a consultant to numerous national and international health care organizations and the pharmaceutical industry. In recent years, Dr Torrance has led or been a major contributor to expert panels that have developed guidelines for the use of economic evaluation in health and medicine for Canada, the United States, and Great Britain. Dr Torrance received the 2001 Award for Career Achievement from the Society for Medical Decision Making and the 2002 President's Award from the International Society for Quality of Life Research.

## Marilyn Dix Smith, RPh, PhD, ISPOR Executive Director

Dr Marilyn Dix Smith is founding trustee and executive director of the International Society for Pharmacoeconomics and Outcomes Research (ISPOR), Lawrenceville, NJ, USA. She serves as chief executive officer of the organization and is responsible for implementing the initiatives of the society. She has extensive experience in the management and financing of scientific organizations.

Dr Smith has designed computer-assisted decision support systems, which compare the costs and clinical outcomes of various disease treatment strategies. Dr Smith has a breadth of experience in disease management, continuous quality improvement, pharmacoeconomic applications, and health care provider and patient education.

Dr Smith was director of professional relations/managed care pharmacy at Lederle Laboratories. Earlier in her career at Lederle, Dr Smith was director of quality control, responsible for product quality testing, operations system design, validation, and compliance. Dr Smith was also production superintendent, where she was responsible for the production of all solid dosage pharmaceutical products.

Dr Smith received her BS in pharmacy and is a registered pharmacist, practicing in community pharmacy. She received her PhD in pharmaceutical science from Ohio State University, and has published many scientific articles, most recently in patient outcomes assessment and pharmacoeconomic analysis. She has authored many professional articles and has given numerous presentations in quality assessment techniques, health care legislation, and disease treatment optimization. Dr Smith was a technical review consultant for the National Cancer Institute and held three 5-year terms on the Committee of Revision, United States Pharmacopoeia. She also was a co-founder of the American Association for Pharmaceutical Scientists, and she is a member of the American Society of Association Executives as well as of many pharmacy and health care organizations.

# Index

**Boldface indicates primary entry.**